ECZEMA HERPETICUM
MY FRIEND THE ENEMY

2nd Edition 2022

by REINHARD HERMES, MS

Table of Contents

Disclaimer

Disclaimer: The information in this book is my personal accounting and history with eczema, herpes, and Eczema Herpeticum. It is not meant to be used, and neither should be utilized to diagnose or treat any medical condition. Please consult your personal physician for diagnosis and/or treatment for any medical problem.

The author is not responsible or liable for any specific health or medical requirements that may arise from any treatment, action, application, or preparation, to any person reading or following the information as outlined in this book. This is strictly my subjective history, and any references provided are for informational purposes only and do not endorse any website or other sources listed in this book.

Also, please be aware that the websites and links in this book may change. They often do. In addition, the author does not have any financial relationship with any source listed in this book. Any names, situations, or details of information are either the authors or changed to protect the privacy of individuals. Thank you for your understanding in these matters

Dedication

I dedicate this book to all "those" whose lives have been affected with Eczema Herpeticum. And while orthodox medicine still has not found a cure for herpes, eczema, or Eczema Herpeticum, other than the use of traditional oral antiviral drugs and topical eczema creams or ointments. Today we have a choice. By opening this book, you've taken that first alternative step *"To Being Eczema and/or Herpes Free."*

Getting back up after we fall is better than going down and staying out. I'm grateful to be part of that effort and wish you the same success that I experienced.

About the Author

Reinhard Hermes, MS, is a Clinical and Community Psychologist whose personal experience and education gives him the expertise to write about Eczema Herpeticum. Born in Berlin, Germany, a naturalized U.S. citizen, he served 4-years in the U.S. Army as a medic in the 46th Medical Battalion, and as an Emergency Room Tech, at Bad Cannstatt 5th General Hospital, Germany. He received his Master of Science degree from California State University, Fullerton. A highly effective and intuitive Psychologist and Nutrition Therapist, he works with clients to achieve maximum health outcomes through personalized consultations. As a strong collaborator, he offers client support through accurate assessments and targeted strategies for the chronically ill.

Competencies include nutritional intervention, Gerson Cancer Therapy, and Emotional Freedom Technique. With strong diagnostic skills, Reinhard participated in several internships that included: Senior Psychometrist at College of Medicine, University of California, Irvine, CA, and the Gerson Training Institute, Cancer Nutrition in San Diego, CA.

Reinhard currently resides in New Market, Maryland and has two grown children who live in California and Nevada. Please contact Reinhard Hermes via email for questions or concerns.

RHermes1@gmail.com

Preface

The doctor has just informed you that the culture came back positive for **Eczema Herpeticum.** What will you tell your husband-bride-to-be? The wedding is next week. In all good stories, books, or motion pictures something always goes wrong.

If nothing goes wrong, there is no movie. The main character doesn't develop. In fact, the worst movies are pulled because they're uninspiring and don't develop. Lots of action, but no depth. That's why there's cable.

In a bad movie the problem or conflict is resolved on some external level. In "Best Picture" films, the main character faces some insurmountable obstacle. Faced with conflict, they grow, change, heal, and develop abilities they didn't have before. And then there are those memorable movies we can watch over-and-over again, because in them the main character also has an internal awakening, reconnecting them with their humanity and community. ***"My Friend, the Enemy"*** *Eczema Herpeticum* is like a movie script; how well you play the part is up to you.

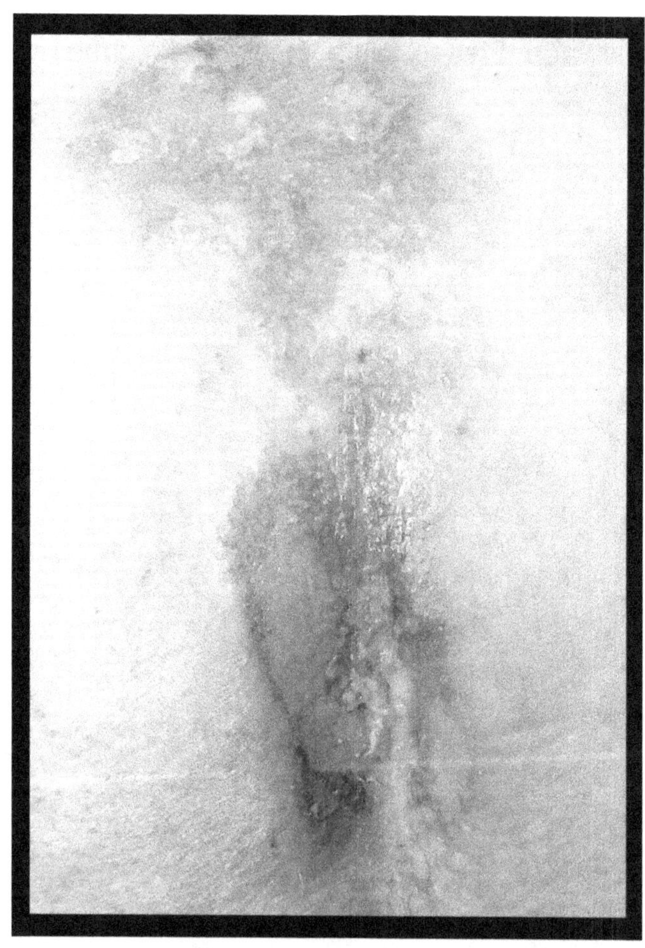

2016 Sacral Eczema Herpeticum

Introduction

"The universe is made of stories, not of atoms."
Muriel Rukeyser (1913 – 1980)

If you've been impacted by **Eczema Herpeticum,** the **Hermes Protocol (HP)** is an account of how I eliminated Genital Herpes infections; thereby removing the threat of Eczema Herpeticum.

There's crucial padding in this manuscript and protocol of eradication. In the past, all the so-called *"herpes or eczema experts"* wanted to get right to the point with easy-to-use procedures that were simple and efficient. The problem? They never worked for me. Getting to the point never stopped herpes or Eczema from their breakout mischief. Part of my healing process was *"patience"* instead of living an abbreviated, infomercial way of life; forever looking for naive solutions or the latest shortcut in a complex world.

Understanding the deception and psychology of COVID-19 or the Russian Ukraine morass can help. As many learned in 2022 the real statistics of COVID were far less dangerous than *"they"* wanted us to believe. But often people don't want to know the truth. It's difficult for some individuals to see beyond the media's storyline or their own beliefs, especially if they've sacrificed health, wealth, family, and future of their children. Some even have been known to be aggressive and cruel towards those who do not buy into the media's narrative. Feeling morally and ethically superior they're inclined to stigmatize, eliminate, and even crush those who do not go along with the *"political-powers-to-be"* irrational narrative. People were physically attacked, and some even killed, simply for not wearing a face mask, which most doctors and scientist knew was a https://bit.ly/3HRCM9I useless prevention strategy in the first place.

Herpes and Eczema can be part of our life situation, but underneath the many physical conditions that make up our life, there exists something deeper and more important. It's called *your life*. Who we truly are. The problem is that we've covered it with so many labels, including Eczema Herpeticum, that we often forget the importance of our *life*. If we could refrain from labeling and mentally identifying with herpes or eczema, then for most these diseases are a physical irritation, discomfort, or minor disability. However, having said that it's important to be properly diagnosed early in the possible complications of Eczema Herpeticum so that an annoyance doesn't turn into an emergency. That's the part we acknowledge. Not the rest of the bunkum and baggage attached to it.

Then instead of the *"Enemy"* using us, we use it to free ourselves from the bondage of unhappiness. Surrendering to our Herpeticum situation in life does not transform its condition; at least not directly. It transforms us. And when we are transformed, our whole world is transformed, because the world reflects the labels and beliefs we attach to it.

Eczema Herpeticum, or with any kind of infection or debility, please *do not feel that you have failed.* Do not feel guilty or blame life for treating you unfairly, but do not blame yourself either. In fact, if anything bad happens in life, use *"the Enemy"* to gain a deeper understanding of who you are. Become an alchemist, transform Herpeticum into healing, and suffering into peace. Be your best *"Friend."* It's uncomplicated with the Hermes Protocol, but I didn't say easy.

Herpeticum has nothing to do with who we are. Whenever any kind of tragedy or misfortune strikes; divorce, illness, disability, loss of job or fortune, break-up of a close relationship, death or suffering of a loved one, know that there is another side to this adversity. You are only steps from transforming the fertilizer of your life into a compost that will bear fruit, and the pain of fear into a jewel of peace.

For most herpes and/or eczema is a physical irritation. Sometimes worse, most of the time just annoying. But for some outbreaks are more than a nuisance. They are a constant threat for emotional disturbances and the risk for more serious **Eczema Herpeticum** complications. What we all have in common is when our mind steps-in and amplifies a nuisance or annoyance into a grievance.

Solutions for Eczema Herpeticum:

1. **Take suppressive** antiviral Medical Prescriptions (Rx) and/or topical Rx eczema creams.

2. **Work with your mind**, and not turn a physical challenge into an emotional delinquent.

3. **Make dietary changes** to support the immune system.

4. **Address candida** and/or systemic fungal infections.

5. **Focus on the immune system** for long-term physical, mental well-being.

Your role in the Hermes Protocol (HP) is to be open to change. **HP** is a two-pronged body-mind approach, to turn the enemy into a long-distance pen-pal and replace frustration with serenity and health.

Hermes Protocol focus:

1. A compromised immune system.
2. Supplements, Vitamins, and Minerals.
3. Candida infection(s).
4. Necessary life-style changes.
5. Long-term emotional answers for peace of mind.

Chronic Herpes or Eczema infections are not a Valtrex or cortisone deficiency. If you're looking for a silver bullet to eliminate herpes and/or eczema outbreaks take the nuclear options: suppressive antiviral pharmaceutical prescription (Rx) drug therapy; topical Rx creams and/or ointments and be done with it. The Hermes Protocol (HP) is about treating symptoms, improving immune function, healing emotions, and supporting the mind. A much healthier, less toxic, and more enduring approach to alleviate outbreaks.

Before we begin, I hope you'll forgive me for mostly using the male pronoun to stand for both genders. Saying he or she over-and-over again is a distraction. Also, please try to resist distress and anxiety when Herpeticum breaks out. Turn away from any mental chatter that says you 'lack.' Run from the inner voice that tells you that you *'fall-short.'* And shut down the *'they win, I lose'* herpes/eczema mental program. Resist your *'outbreak-brains'* negative chatter by sifting it through a filter of realism. Live less serious, not by ignoring the facts-of-life, but by putting the past behind you.

Like Shakespeare said, *"I would rather have a fool make me merry, than experience make me sad."* Accept the reality that peace of mind is moment-by-moment and day-to-day effort. Also, there are numerous hyperlinks in this book for validating information. That's the good and bad news, because they can also be a distraction. In addition, and as you know the internet is a fluid and changing environment; therefore, some links may be broken. Thank you for your patience and understanding.

I want to thank you for buying **My Friend, The Enemy: Eczema Herpeticum**. The second book in the **My Friend, the Enemy** series. **Genital Herpes** was the first and is an in-depth examination detailing herpes history and protocols to eliminate outbreaks. This book includes a condensed *herpes* version but with a focus on eczema and Herpeticum. My suggestion is that you may also want to read Genital Herpes to get a deeper understanding on how to eliminate herpes outbreaks. Thank you for your consideration, Reinhard Hermes.

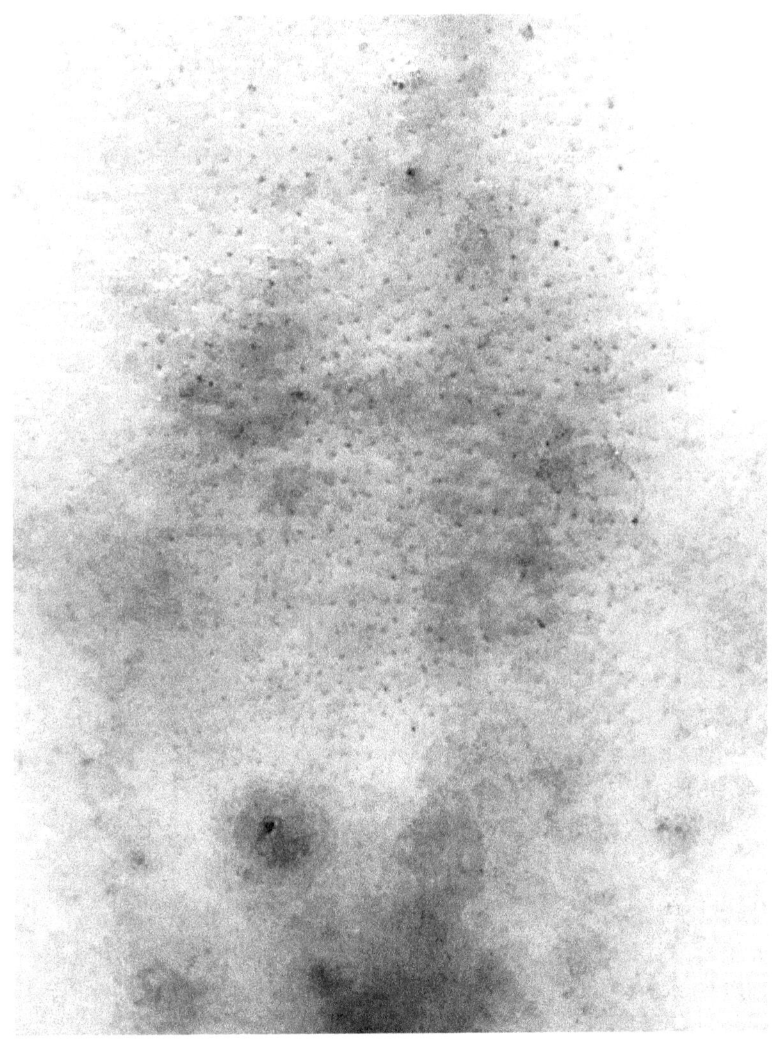

2016 Eczema Herpeticum Outbreak

Chapter 1: Infections

"When all else fails, take a Rx for lighthearted humor.
It's the best medicine for suffering." – RH

A couple of herpes infections a year was not a big deal. However, in time their frequency and severity increased, and in 2016 reached hurricane crescendo with more than 70 Genital Herpes outbreaks, including a severe and serious complication of **Eczema Herpeticum.** It even concerned my stoic doctors. Eczema Herpeticum outbreaks persisted from October 2016 to April 2017, but as of June 2022 I've been Genital Herpes and Eczema Herpeticum outbreak free. Most often eczema and herpes are two distinct mostly harmless diseases but combined they potentially spell *'danger'* if not dealt with promptly.

Eczema Herpeticum is an infection where the herpes viral hunter enlists eczema to do its mischief. Like a full-blown hurricane, with its distorted pain, sacral or facial discomfort, turbulent nights, but the outbreaks paled compared to the anxiety I experienced when I "Googled" Eczema Herpeticum.

Herpeticum and my emotional response was certainly a part of the reason my wife and I divorced. However, if my experience will resonate and help someone put herpes and/or eczema in remission, and a smile back on their face, then my experience will not have been pointless or in vain.

Your goal is to eliminate herpes infections and/or eczema rashes. This book is focused on eliminating herpes outbreaks; thereby, eliminating or minimizing the chance of getting an Eczema Herpeticum infection. The other approach is to eliminate eczema rashes, and we go over that process as well. Even though I've eliminated herpes and Eczema Herpeticum outbreaks, I occasionally still get an eczema rash on my sacrum if I deviate from my diet and eat too many carbohydrates and sugar.

A. Eczema

Eczema, also commonly termed Atopic Dermatitis, is a chronic skin disease that causes itchiness, dry, irritated, red, inflamed skin. It often starts in early childhood and if not controlled can last a lifetime. Although it can affect the entire body, it's usually found on the scalp, cheeks, chin, back, legs, elbows, and arms. High perspiration areas, creases of the elbows, knees, hands, and feet are frequently affected. Moderate to severe itching is a common characteristic at any age.

Eczema may go through periods of healing, or remission, when there are almost no symptoms. However, it can become aggravated, and then symptoms worsen. This is known as a flare-up. People with eczema are often advised to avoid triggers, situations that may cause eczema outbreaks.

Triggers are different for each person and can include:

1. Eggs, dairy products, soy, chocolate, peanuts (keep a journal).
2. Specific soaps and detergents.
3. Dry cleaning clothes (cleaning fluids are very toxic).
4. Fragrances.
5. Nail polish.
6. Allergens.
7. Stress aggravates eczema.
8. Certain foods, gluten in wheat, oats, rye, and barley.
9. Other irritants or allergens.
10. A dangerous trigger, Herpes Simplex Virus.

Most eczema outbreaks heal without long-term problems. However, sometimes eczema becomes infected. Typically, this happens when a fungus, bacteria, or virus gets into the rash. These are commonly caused by *"scratching the itch."* Scratching opens the skin and makes it vulnerable to infections. The more you scratch, the worse eczema becomes and the longer it takes to heal. Excess or lack of humidity promotes itching. Overbathing and showering and using harsh soaps can contribute to skin dryness, causing more itching. Use a mild, moisturizing soap, and bath oil. Apply moisturizers (coconut oil worked well for the author) frequently, especially after showering.

It's important to know what causes your eczema outbreak to become infected, its signs, symptoms, and available treatment options. The following are some of the more common microbes responsible for causing eczema infections:

1. Staphylococcus aureus (Staph infection)
2. Fungal infections, such as ringworm (Tinea)
3. Herpes simplex virus (HSV-1 or HSV-2)

Staphylococcus Aureus is a type of bacteria found on the skin of most people with eczema. It also lives on the skin of about 20 percent of healthy adults. *Staphylococcus aureus* thrives on weeping or broken skin. In cases of a staph infection, eczema spreads more quickly and makes healing difficult. If left untreated, an eczema staph infection may cause a blood infection known as *sepsis* which can be fatal if not treated promptly. In general, the younger the person, the more likely they are to develop complications from an infection. Infants and young children are at particular risk of developing blood or bacterial infections, so a doctor should examine them as soon as possible.

Ringworm is a common source of fungal infections in eczema. Ringworm can be found all over the body and typically appears as isolated patches. It often occurs between the toes, where it is known as athlete's foot. Fungal infections are more likely to occur in people with eczema, but they are relatively common in all individuals.

Herpes is the one exception, which can cause serious or even fatal complications for those with eczema, either **Cold Sores HSV-1 or Genital Herpes HSV-2.** It's best for people with eczema to avoid individuals with active Cold Sores or Genital Herpes. Most people with eczema experience clearing in their late twenties, and by age 30 many are in remission of the disease; although, a minority develop chronic localization in their hands, known as hand dermatitis (Below: 2016 Sacral Eczema Herpeticum Infection).

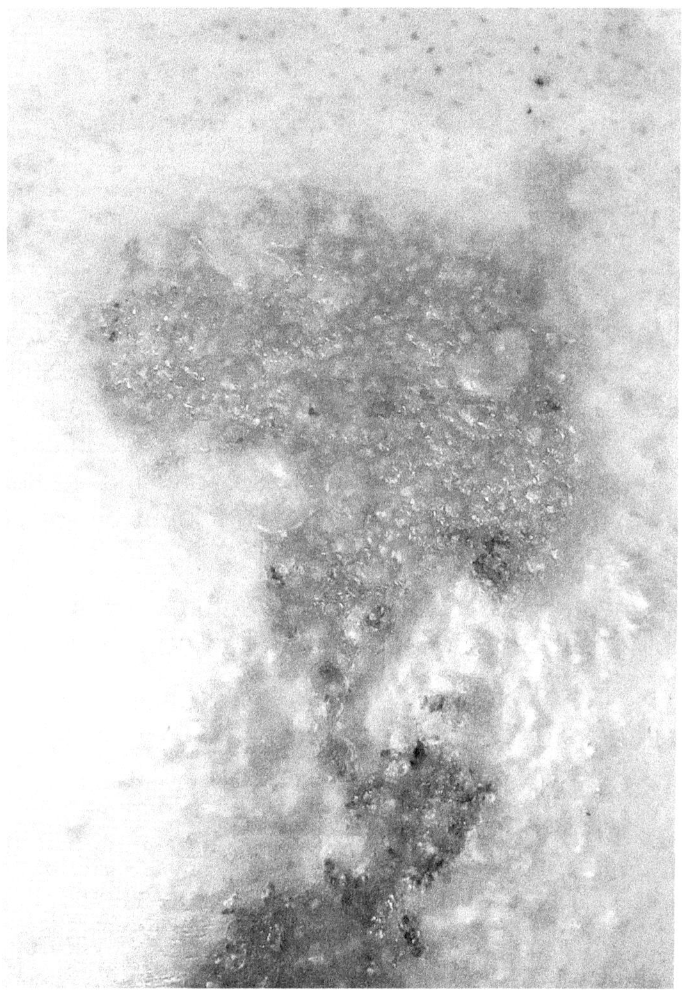

B. Herpes

According to Wikipedia *"herpesviridae"* is a large family of DNA viruses. They are also known as herpesviruses, derived from the Greek word *herpein, or "to creep."* As in recurring outbreaks or infections give me the *"creeps."* In total, there are about 130 herpes viruses. Most are found in mammals, birds, fish, reptiles, amphibians, and mollusks http://bit.ly/2DVWCIWiki.

Depending on your source, 90% of U.S. adults are infected with at least one of these:

1. HSV-1, Cold Sores, typically occur around the mouth, lips, or face.
2. HSV-2, can involve the labia, genitals, sacrum, buttocks, and anus.
3. Varicella zoster virus, chickenpox, and shingles.
4. Epstein-Barr virus, implicated in mononucleosis.
5. Cytomegalovirus.
6. Human papillomavirus (HPV).

A bigger problem than making sense of herpes statistics is that most people (85%) don't know they're infected. They've never been symptomatic.

How to prevent getting infected with herpes. It's difficult. As human beings we make human contact. There are steps we can take to reduce the risk, but at some point, somewhere, by someone, nearly everyone gets infected. To help prevent the spread of Genital Herpes avoid all sexual contact during an outbreak. Always use condoms. It's not a guarantee, just like an auto umbrella insurance policy is not a guarantee against getting into an accident. But no matter what, don't drive without a condom.

It doesn't seem to matter anymore whether you're infected with HSV-1 or HSV-2. The Hermes Protocol is effective for both. The contamination risk for the other partner is the same. Anyone infected with HSV of either type can transmit HSV to their partner at any time if those parts make contact.

During an initial infection, the herpes virus replicates in cell after cell at the point of origin. Like any living organism, its purpose is to reproduce and spread. Immediately, the immune system responds. A fierce battle starts, which can manifest itself as an "outbreak." Herpes functions by taking over a living cell. That cell becomes a viral host. To deactivate the virus, our immune system kills the cell and the virus. Like guerilla warfare, the herpes virus escapes the immune system by traveling up nerve fibers to an area known as ganglia. In effect, it hides out, and viral replication ceases. Herpes is then considered *"dormant."*

Herpes uses a **"Star-Wars"** cloaking maneuver to avoid discovery and annihilation. The immune system can't *"see"* the virus while it's dormant. For those with a strong and vigilant immune system, herpes can stay hidden for years and then break out when we're *"run-down"* or immune compromised. People with healthy immune systems often don't know they're infected.

Initial warning signs, whether HSV-2 or HSV-1, of Genital Herpes symptoms are not much different from those of Cold Sores. They can differ from person to person but are more complex for females.

Symptoms:

1. **HSV-2 blisters** on and around the genital area, rectum, inner thighs, and buttocks.
2. **In women,** blister can also arise in the cervix and discharge from the vagina.
3. **Urinary Tract** Infections.

4. **Pain** when urinating for both genders.
5. **HSV-1** blisters around the mouth, nose, underneath the chin.
6. **Flu-like symptoms,** with fever, chills, shooting pains, muscle aches.
7. **Infections** normally last about two weeks.
8. **Doctors** generally treat HSV-1 or HSV-2 with antiviral medication.

See your health care provider ASAP if you experience any rash or strange infection to *"test"* if it's herpes.

Triggers & Stages

Prodromal Stage: during the first herpes outbreak (prodromal stage), small clusters of white blisters may occur. The blisters break and leave tender sores. Other symptoms include pain, fever, itching, burning, and swelling of the lymph nodes in the groin area.

Asymptomatic stage: the herpes virus lies dormant in nerve cells. At times it can reactivate and move to the surface of the skin without causing any symptoms. Herpes can be transmitted even if there are no visible symptoms. It's called asymptomatic viral shedding. For most who live with herpes it's a nonevent. For some it's a nuisance. But for a minority, their lives are dramatized and often exaggerated by chronic outbreaks, skin complications like Eczema Herpeticum, and emotional complexities.

Outbreak Triggers:

1. Alcohol
2. General illness
3. Dehydration
4. Emotional stress
5. Fatigue
6. Immune Compromised
7. Medications, chemotherapy, AIDS.
7. Low immunity
8. Menstruation
9. Poor nutrition
10. Physical stress
11. Excessive Sunlight
12. Physical trauma to affected area.

Unfortunately, the Genital Herpes stigma is not getting better. Maybe over-spinning the hysteria pendulum of Genital Herpes is not such a bad thing. The *"madness"* is like a collective over-dramatized ego phenomenon. And like all ego shooting fuzzballs, they burn up when they enter the atmosphere of reality. A problem with the Genital Herpes health dilemma is that most pain inflicted by the herpes virus is not *physical, but emotional.* Having said that, please remember there is a silent minority who suffer debilitating, and at times, life threating physical symptoms that can be both emotionally draining and physically challenging.

Cold Sores, AKA Fever Blisters: typically appear outside the mouth, under the nose, around the lips, or underneath the chin. OK, so we get a cold sore. How bad can it be? As it turns out, **HSV-1** can be more troublesome than our HSV-2 sexual predator. Since HSV-1 involves mostly facial nerve cells, it can spread to the eyes, causing **Ocular Herpes**, which can result in blindness.

In fact, Ocular Herpes is the most common cause of blindness in the industrial world, with over 500,000 cases reported each year in the U.S. alone. So, primp up, put in those contacts. *Sorry, not with those fingers.* Wash your hands first (and thoroughly) before putting in your contacts. No matter what. Even if you don't think you have an active outbreak. HSV-1 has also been known to infect the brain, creating a condition known as Herpes-Simplex-Encephalitis (HSE). It has a mortality rate of up to 30% with anti-vital treatment and 70-80% without treatment. When death happens, it's usually because of severe inflammation and brain swelling. Both conditions are a grim reminder if we're careless with HSV-1.

Historically HSV-1 indicated oral herpes, while HSV-2 signified genital outbreaks. Due to the prevalence of oral sex, the location of outbreaks is no longer a reliable indicator. In fact, HSV-1 is increasingly found on genital cultures. A quick reminder: if you have Cold Sores (HSV-1), it does NOT protect you from Genital Herpes (HSV-2), which is why most people have both.

Canker Sores

There seems to be some confusion regarding **Cold Sores vs. Canker Sores.** Cold Sores are herpes lesions. Canker sores are not. They are aphthous ulcers. Small, shallow sores found inside the mouth or at the base of the gums.

Canker Sores (Aphthous Ulcers) are painful but benign sores that occur on the tongue, inside the lips, cheeks, gums, or palate. There's no evidence that canker sores are caused by a virus or any infectious agent. However, they're common and often confused with mouth infections. They heal without treatment, but an array of over-the-counter products help ease their pain. Like herpes, there's no magic pill to prevent or cure canker sores. The good news, the Hermes Protocol helps all virus-related infections.

I'm not a doctor. This book is my experience and not a substitute for seeing one. *Acyclovir* is recognized as the first line of Rx defense and treatment of choice for herpes. Don't resist taking it, especially if there is pain or difficulty urinating. Antiviral prescriptions (Rx) are expensive, and they may not be covered by insurance. Make sure your doctor or pharmacist knows generic brand options. Wal-Mart pharmacies are often a cost-effective choice. If uninsured, Planned Parenthood is an alternative. For more information contact Planned Parenthood at (800) 230-7526.

Traditional pharmaceutical antivirals can be taken daily and make it less likely (but not guaranteed) to pass the infection to your partner(s). Mainstream medicine's standard of care are antivirals, such as Acyclovir or Valtrex. They have been known to:

1. Sometimes eliminate outbreaks entirely.
2. Diminish them to a rare occurrence.
3. Alleviate suffering greatly.

Their downside: certain individuals carry a great deal of risk for serious complications. Taking them depends on your risk-reward threshold. They did not work well for the author because of their side effects. To give the body a fighting chance against a formidable foe, start with lifestyle choices. Yes, there's that dirty word again. *Lifestyle*. A long-winded acronym for *"No fun, no way!"*

Lifestyle for many is the most difficult part of the Hermes Protocol. Like asking an alcoholic to drink Perrier at Happy Hour. Or a one-armed, Facebook, iPhone tweeting junky to handwrite a letter. I've heard it said it's easier to change a person's religion than their lifestyle. I guess it depends on how much suffering we can take.

When herpes infections occur, start looking for some possible connections between stress, food allergies, alcohol, sun exposure, medications, constipation, or any other variable that activates outbreaks. Topicals help, but they're like pulling out the smoke alarm to douse a fire. It may drown out the noise, but it won't do much to extinguish the flames. Herpes is the fire alarm, a blinking red light in the immune system's dashboard. It's warning us to slow down, change our way, or stop. *"Danger, Will Robinson, danger."* Life is too stressful, and the body has been pushed beyond its immune limits.

A 'positive' exception to a sudden increase in outbreaks can be a *"healing crisis."* For example, starting an antiviral like Valtrex, the body has more ammunition. Herpes fights back, increases its viral shedding, and more outbreaks occur. A healing crisis is beneficial, and not a regression of well-being. The difficult part is differentiating between a beneficial healing crisis or a regression occurrence.

Antiviral Medications

1. Acyclovir (Sitavig, Zovirax) is the oldest of the four antiviral drugs. It inhibits herpes by disrupting its DNA replication and comes in a variety of application methods, including pill form and ointment. I was prescribed Acyclovir for Genital Herpes with these instructions:

Initial Acyclovir treatment for Genital Herpes was 200 mg by mouth every four hours while awake (five times daily) for 10 days, or 400 mg every eight hours for 7-10 days.

Intermittent treatment for recurrences was 200 mg by mouth every four hours while awake (five times daily) for five days. To be started at the earliest sign of symptoms.

Chronic suppression for recurrence was 400 mg by mouth every 12 hours for up to 12 months, or 200 mg three to five times daily. The author was NOT able to continue suppressive therapy because of acute side effects. Found myself in the ER on too many occasions with skyrocketing blood pressure (kidneys).

2. Valtrex (Valacyclovir) Valtrex common side effects include headaches, nausea, stomach pain, vomiting, and dizziness. It's the antiviral commercial that features happy looking couples who are just a bit too cheerful about their herpes diagnoses.

3. Famvir (Famciclovir) Famvir is an antiviral that can slow the spread of herpes symptoms. It's especially useful for Herpes Zoster (shingles), strong herpes outbreaks, and a suppressed immune system because of HIV. It seems less toxic based on the potency of side effects.

Every Day or As Needed

Choosing *"Every Day or As Needed"* is not like deciding what socks to wear with what shoes. I don't think twice about taking a daily multi-vitamin. Taking daily "suppressive" antiviral therapy rings different today. But only because I experienced terrible side effects and got tired of going to the Emergency Room. All medications have some inherent safety risks. Although antivirals are generally well tolerated, the internet is littered with unfortunate souls who found out too late to be cautious when taking any medication. No matter what your doctor or anyone else tells you--be cautious. Above all, be extremely careful if you have any kidney or liver issues.

Risks & Side Effects

All medications have risks. Most who take antiviral medication have few side effects, or minor ones. The most common are:

1. Feeling sick and nauseous,
2. Vomiting,
3. Diarrhea and/or abdominal pain,
4. Breaking out in skin rashes,
5. Including photosensitivity, and
6. Itching.

Some have more serious reactions. Then there are those with liver or kidney disease, who probably should not take antivirals unless it's an absolute life and death situation. Inadequate hydration increases the chances for kidney failure. Drink plenty of water to stay well hydrated when taking antivirals. Early warning signs of kidney problems include decreased urination and kidney flank pain. Kidney pain often feels like lower back pain. Other symptoms include loss of appetite, difficulty thinking clearly, dizziness, headaches, metallic taste in your mouth, fatigue, and itchiness.

Valtrex (approved 1995) http://bit.ly/2BzYnjn and Acyclovir (approved 1982) can cause liver damage in some patients. Signs of liver inflammation include yellowing of the skin and eyes. The elderly, and those with a compromised immune system, may not tolerate Valtrex. Please tell your doctor if you have kidney or liver problems before taking any medication.

Technical Abstracts and Studies

1. Acyclovir Studies http://bit.ly/2rHWIZk
2. Valtrex Studies http://bit.ly/2BAnVNl
3. Herpes Simplex Virus http://bit.ly/2niNQEY

Valtrex is often prescribed for long-term (months or years) suppression of HSV outbreaks. Valtrex has been involved with over 10,000 patients in clinical trials of up to one year in duration. There is considerable confidence in its long-term safety at doses up to 1000 mg/day.

Acyclovir, on the other hand, has been evaluated for 10 years in a wide range of patients with recurrent Genital Herpes infections. To date, resistance to Acyclovir is rare. The effectiveness and safety of Acyclovir and Valtrex are maintained even when used long term, or acute treatment over many years.

Famcyclovir (Famvir, approved 1997) is the newest member of the three *virusketeers*. From observational and anecdotal reports, Famvir is well tolerated. Currently, there are no known "severe" side effects. However, it should be noted there are also no long-term studies. Therefore, its side effects may not be fully known. The most serious Famvir risk is an allergic reaction: http://bit.ly/2DVvZgE

Famvir is also eliminated through the kidneys. Those with impaired kidney or liver function should be cautious and consider taking a lower dose. Patients with liver damage are advised against taking Famvir or be very cautious!

Chapter 2: You Survived

"Divine wisdom does not judge, criticize, or condemn. It gets even." – RH

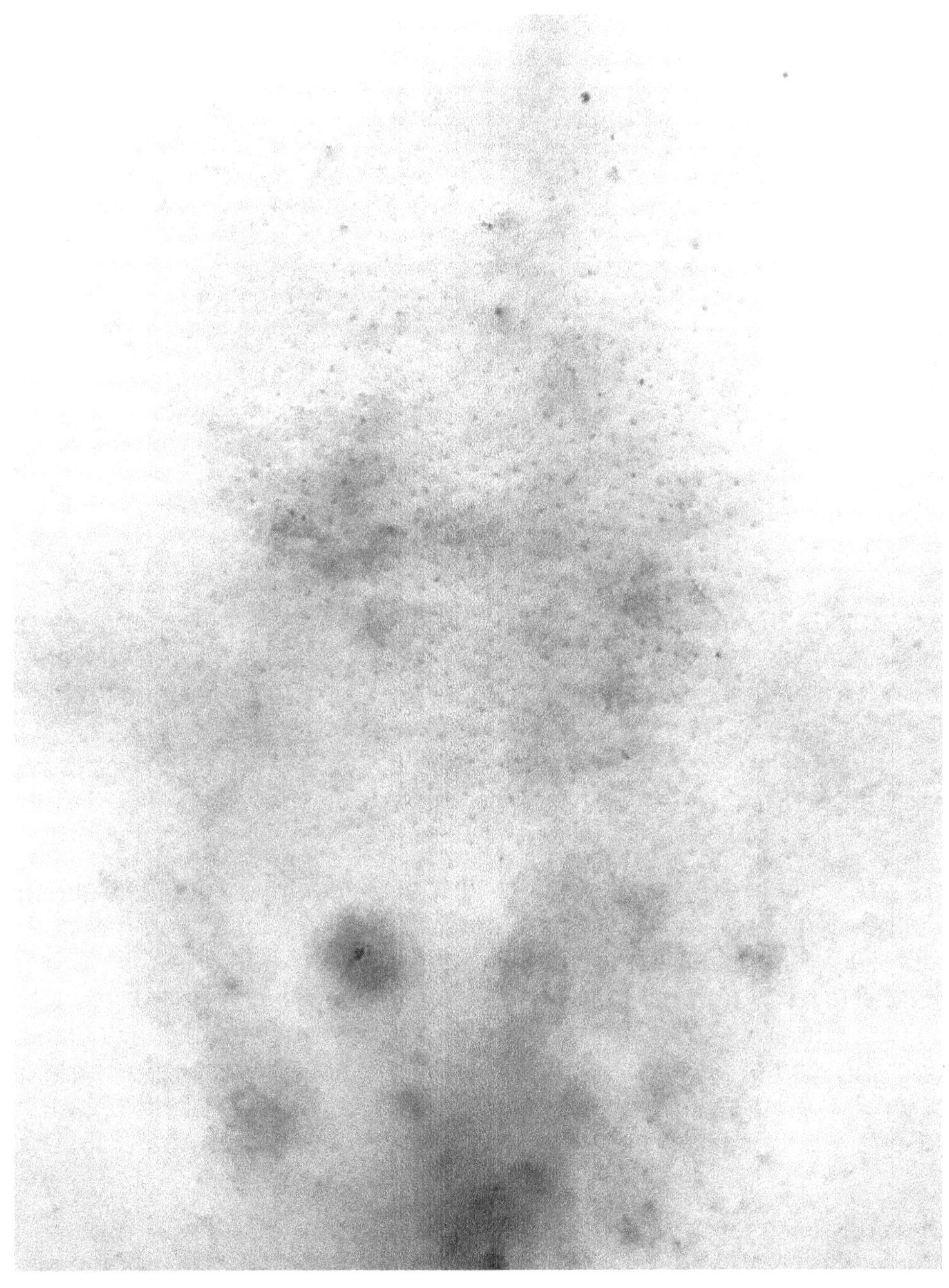

2016 Sacral Eczema Herpeticum

A. Eczema Herpeticum

Before 2015, Genital Herpes was just inconvenient and emotionally draining. That changed with my first eczema flare-up. I had no idea how troublesome eczema can be for those infected with the herpes virus. (See Photo Above: 2016 Sacral Eczema Herpeticum Outbreak)

With eczema there are potential triggers that make symptoms worse. What is relatively unknown is that one of the most dangerous trigger is herpes. Either Cold Sores or Genital Herpes. Who knew? My general practitioner (GP) never said a word. Most GPs are unfamiliar with the complications of having eczema and herpes break out in the same location, at the same time. They don't see it enough. It's more in the realm of textbook dermatology or infectious disease. Please be vigilant if you're infected with both herpes and eczema. Eczema Herpeticum can be a disaster, waiting for a train wreck.

Eczema Herpeticum (EH) develops when eczema-damaged skin is infected with the Herpes Simplex Virus HSV-1 or HSV- 2. A herpes infection on an Eczematous area of the skin can quickly spread into a painful, blistery, oozing rash. Like an out-of-control brush fire, if left untreated it can spread to vital organs throughout the body. On rare occasions it is still fatal. It was October 2016 when Genital Herpes and eczema turned unpleasant for the author.

B. Negativity Bias

One of the first things to realize about your Eczema Herpeticum experience and trauma is *"You survived."* Acknowledging ***"I survived"*** can be a news flash to the psyche and nervous system. That's not to imply that we try to convince ourselves that Herpeticum is a blessing or a gift, but to think of it as a "given." It makes it *easier not to rationalize or blame* outbreak frustrations on anyone else. If something is a *given*, it just is. Don't deny or pretend herpes or eczema doesn't exist. Start by acknowledging them, then have the best life possible going forward.

That's not always easy in an age of blame and shame, contrived effects, and social isolation. The concept of healing our pain and treating ourselves with compassion has gotten a bad rap. Conformist moral thinking goes something like this. *"Loving ourselves is narcissistic, selfish, self-indulgent, and the supreme fantasy of a disguised ego looking out for number one."* I don't speak French, but I know a few German words, and my answer to that ridiculous notion is, *"Bullshit!"* Ooops, that's not German, that's Houston. In fact, if we have a chronic disease, like herpes or eczema, the opposite is true. If the airplane cabin pressure dropped on the way to San Jose, no one would call us selfish if we secured our oxygen mask first before helping another.

No matter what the disease or outer circumstance, to honor oneself is to come into harmony with life itself, including our family, friends, and everyone else. For most of us, our experiences are usually a mixed basket of both positive and negative events. But scientists who study human behavior tell us that we have a *'negativity-bias.'* It makes us especially alert to danger and threat.

Because of this negativity-bias, we can feel lost or discouraged from chronic eczema outbreaks and/or herpes infections and difficult to evoke positive memories, feelings of joy, and comfort.

Yes, herpes and/or eczema can be serious and debilitating. But while enduring the healing process, don't forget to live. Being Herpeticum "free" is a process, not a switch. Don't put life on hold or keep mourning the loss of your *Life Before Herpeticum* **(LBH)**. The consequences can be more detrimental than outbreaks. A saner approach to life is to have an attitude of honoring things, but not making them *so important.* Maintaining a feeling of *glad to be alive yet* acknowledging Herpeticum outbreaks with an open mind. That doesn't mean we sit back and do nothing. We stay proactive about taking the necessary steps to be "Herpes-Free." We don't belittle or make light of our problems, but neither do we fan them into an inferno of *"big-deals."*

C. Immune System

Returning to well-being with the **Hermes Protocol** by addressing the immune system, nutrition, diet, supplementation, lifestyle changes, mindfulness, and detoxification. Given the right conditions, the body can restore itself to a state of dynamic equilibrium called *"good-health."*

From eczema flare-ups to herpes outbreaks, to Eczema Herpeticum infections, the Hermes Protocol (HP) set me "Free." My prison-break-strategy worked. I've been on outbreak and infection parole since May 2017. Maybe the Hermes Protocol can transform your negativity bias and grant you freedom?

IMPORTANT: Many people keep looking and hoping to find a "by-the-numbers" cure: do these six steps and *"no-more-herpes-or-eczema."* There is a simpler way. Remember my suggestion? It's simple. Take suppressive antiviral therapy and/or topical steroid creams. If it works, great! It didn't for me.

Herpeticum freedom is independence from a lifestyle that compromises our immune system. Without herpes outbreaks there is no Herpeticum, only an occasional eczema rash. Remember, the primary focus of this book is to eliminate herpes outbreaks; thereby, eliminating Eczema Herpeticum. Look at the Hermes Protocol with a deeper "understanding." Not a cursory skimming. There is no shortcut answer. In fact, I know of only one treatment for Herpeticum that works 100% of the time. Not getting infected with the herpes virus in the first place.

D. Out of Love

"Raise your words, not voice.
It is rain that grows flowers, not thunder." – Rumi

In life's unpredictable journey, Genital Herpes and eczema often separates us from loved ones. If Herpeticum gets between you, don't let outbreaks isolate you further from society. Eczema Herpeticum played a part in losing my marriage. Like any health crisis that demands our constant attention, it's a price many pay when challenged with a chronic disease. But working the Hermes Protocol, you'll re-discover who you are. Feelings of loneliness, grief, and guilt can turn into appreciation, self-worth, and contentment.

Of all the "self-help" books, novels, or movies seen, none has ever approached the feelings of awe and wonder of *"falling in love."* Or the despair and pain of falling out-of-love. That is life.

If or when they occur, heartbreak and/or Herpeticum, our Grecian mask of cynicism is there to hide the heartbreak of grief. In those wounded moments, a cynical heart can seem like the best defense. But before giving up and rejecting love as a personal illusion, feeling it takes more than it gives, finish the Hermes Protocol.

Eczema and herpes are only two of many reasons for the collapse of many traditional social interactions and values. For men, blasted with a constant barrage of #Me-Too negativity and fear mongering by the media, we compound the problem by avoidance and escaping vis-a-vis our addictive quest for "more-and-more" pleasure instead of seeking real and lasting happiness. There are easier ways to achieve happiness that are free, as opposed to fleeting pleasures that often carry a steep price of addiction and despair. Continue reading to find out more.

Relationships

Eczema and/or herpes can affect every aspect of life. Whether single, married, or in a committed relationship, each person responds to disease in their own way, depending on their experience with illness, familial history, personal values, psychological makeup, finances, or health insurance. Or whether they live alone or as a couple.

While herpetic infections or eczema flare-ups often raise questions and issues for the infected person. Partners are also faced with their own challenges. And depending on the frequency and severity of symptoms, unwelcome thoughts can creep into a partner's consciousness:

1. *"Should I stay or cut my losses and go?*
2. *"What about our sex life?"*
3. *"What do I do when there isn't any?"*
4. *"Then what happens to our intimacy?"*
5. *"Will our relationship ever feel the same again?"*
6. *"I'm scared that I might get infected."*

When diagnosed with Eczema Herpeticum most people are forced to navigate through unchartered territory. Not only with medical uncertainty but with coming to terms with a current or future relationship. If you are in a committed relationship, you might be staring into a foggy future of solitude. There is anguish in losing spontaneous intimacy. It will test the level of your resilience with the person you love most. Or examine the shallowness of forgiveness in yourself or your partner.

Love between two people is never simple. But none more complicated than when there is a third or even a fourth party involved: Eczema, Cold Sores, Genital Herpes, and/or Eczema Herpeticum. We pretend to know what love is. Talk about it lightly. Seldom acknowledging how powerful and lasting its currents are. We expect it to be healing and whole, even when faced with a chronic disease. Then we are astonished to find that love at times is frail and human, affecting division in relationships and failures in marriages.

Let me ask you a question? Would you marry the love of your life if they were breaking out with Genital Herpes every 10 days, eczema flare-ups every 2 months, or a super Eczema Herpeticum infection every 6 months? What's the cut-off? I mean, what kind of honeymoon lovefest are we talking about? It never occurred to me or my wife "for worse" or "in sickness" would turn into a constant outbreak emotional roller-coaster marathon, including a nasty Eczema Herpeticum obstacle course. Knowing what we know today, I'm sure neither would've committed to such an ordeal. But then the "for worse" only happens to the "others" on the 6 o'clock news, not us *decent* folks.

Life doesn't always go according to our delusions. One day, within our mundane turbulence of going to work, coming home and grocery shopping, and doing a week's worth of laundry, something happens that you didn't count on. You have a Genital Herpes outbreak. Two weeks later you have an eczema rash appear on your sacrum. Then another, and another. And they just keep coming, until one day they combine into a super infection, Eczema Herpeticum.

For couples, nonstop eczema rashes or herpes infections with their Herpeticum complications are not just a diversion of single solitaire, but a 24-7 game of war. Without any victor. When one partner is infected, both lives are interrupted. Like any chronic illness, Eczema Herpeticum disrupts day-to-day routines and life's familiar patterns. It forces relationships to dig deeper. Many times, to their bedrock, having to make decisions that were unthinkable just a year before. By the way, *"Mr. Herpeticum, I had my fingers crossed when I spoke those vows."* The disease process is easier with a strong supportive partner, rather than being in the late stages of a tired, weathered relationship. But statistics or demographics seldom determine who gets well and who continues to suffer.

We come to realize some couples stay together, while others fall apart and get divorced. It's nobody's fault but a learning period for both partners. Yes, there may be grief and pain. But only because we want to cling and hang on to something that's no longer there. There is never any justification for revenge or anger. No matter what the other person did or didn't do. We accept them and move on. That's the only way we'll ever change in a positive way and have any chance at future happiness. This is often a difficult concept to accept. We're so used to seeing the world through our shame & blame "justified-anger-revenge" bifocals. Black or white, right, or wrong, and good or bad. But like pleasure, it doesn't lead to happiness. *"The most important step out the karmic law is forgiveness."* Eckhart Tolle

Words of Love

We can't control what happens in life, but we can control our response. And that's important. Create something out of your Herpeticum experience. Even if the relationship falls apart. Make use of it. Whether we're rich or poor, win the lottery or lose everything, infected with Herpeticum, diagnosed with cancer, or healthy. Those are the ingredients of life. They are sometimes the problem but seldom the dilemma.

It's our relationship to them that causes us more difficulties. If our relationship isn't working, we call it growing pains, or misery. But it's plain old suffering. So, if we get divorced, we'll be rid of our marriage pain. Replacing it with being alone and single person's pain. We've changed one ingredient for another.

The "real" problem has not disappeared. It's only changed its shape and form. If we can realize that, maybe we can stop the fantasy. *"Once I find the perfect partner everything will be OK." They're not out there.* It's the belief that once I change my "situation," quit my job, exchange my husband, live by myself, stop drinking, and be Herpeticum free, then I'll be happy. Good luck.

Chapter 3: Getting Tested

A. Herpes Diagnosis

It's best to diagnose herpes at the first sign of a lesion. Get examined ASAP by a doctor if there are unusual sores, a smelly discharge, burning sensation when urinating, or bleeding for women between periods. A physician can often diagnose herpes by noting and looking at a person's symptoms. But a culture is highly recommended. It will give a definitive diagnosis.

Once a lesions crusts over it has poor accuracy. If the window of opportunity is missed, repeat the culture at the beginning of the next outbreak. Choose one of several options listed below. There are other skin conditions that can mimic a herpes infection: *Eczema, Lichen Sclerosis, Syphilis, Molluscum Contagiosum, Impetigo, and Yeast Infections.* Get tested to make sure it's herpes (HSV).

According to the *American Sexual Health Association* **(ASHA)** "…there are different tests available for herpes. Viral culture and DNA tests can be done if you are experiencing symptoms. Blood tests are available for people who may not have symptoms or if the signs have already healed." http://bit.ly/2DGThDD

Herpes Viral Lesions Test

If a Genital Herpes outbreak occurs, take a viral culture or a swab test within the first 48 hours of onset. It takes about a week to get results. According to ASHA, the **herpes viral culture** test has a major pro and con. The test is known for its accuracy. If your test results are positive for herpes, rest insecure. You have the virus.

Also, the test identifies whether a person is infected with the HSV-1 or HSV-2 virus. However, the viral culture test needs an active virus. If the lesion has started to crust, there's a good chance of not getting an accurate reading.

NAAT Test

Apart from a swab test, a *Nucleic Acid Amplification Testing* **(NAAT)** can also check for herpes. Because of speed and accuracy, and its lower risk for a false negative, NAATs are the preferred method of testing. The most common NAAT method is the *Polymerase Chain Reaction* or **PCR** test. The test is performed on cells or fluids from a sore and/or blood or other bodily fluids.

PCR tests are known for their accuracy and a 4-hour quick turnaround. The downside, they're expensive and not yet widely available.

Antibody or Blood Test

Doctors can perform an antibody or blood test to determine if a person is infected with the herpes virus even before an outbreak occurs. The test searches for immunoglobulin (IgG) antibodies in the blood. It also verifies whether it's HSV-1 or HSV-2.

The antibody test is known for its accuracy. The timeframe when the IgG antibodies can be detected varies from person to person. Some have detectable IgG antibody levels in weeks, others in months. There's a good chance the test will yield a false negative if a person tests too soon. ASHA advises waiting 12 to 16 weeks after exposure to ensure that antibodies can be detected. (See Below: 2016_11_09 Sacral Eczema Herpeticum)

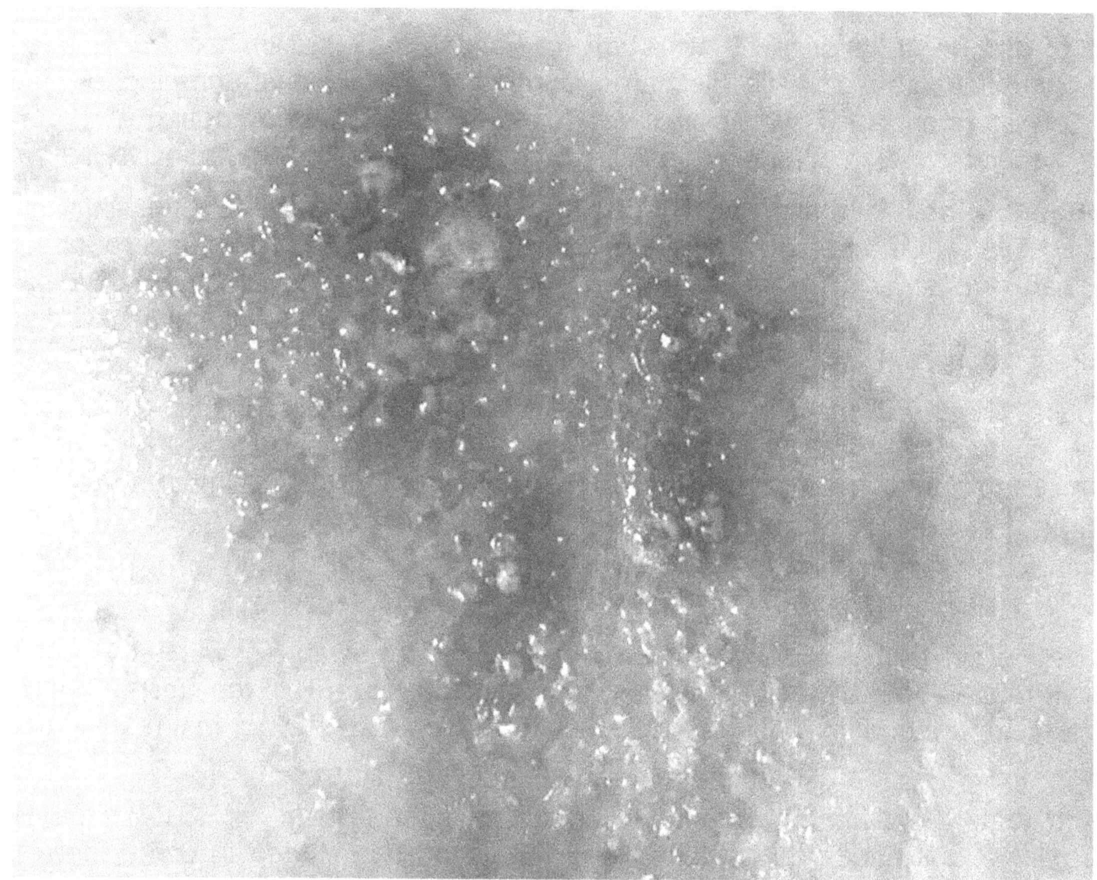

B. Not Getting Infected

The secret to not getting infected with Genital Herpes is to live like David Vetter. Affectionately known as the "boy in the bubble," David was born in 1971 with Severe Combined Immune Deficiency (SCID). For 12 years David captured our attention as he lived in a sterilized dome to maintain a germ-free environment. herpes probably would have killed David. Few of us are capable or willing to isolate like David Vetter just to avoid herpes. The reality is we don't have to. Most of us already have some form of the virus. http://bit.ly/2DFWvYb

Herpes sheds about 10 percent of the time without an outbreak, according to a recent study published in the *Journal of American Medical Association*. It matters little if the other person has symptoms or not. We can still get infected. http://bit.ly/2rQlSVY With an active outbreak, try not to touch the sores or their fluids. Herpes can be transferred to other parts of your body. Be especially careful around the eyes (Ocular Herpes) and people you come in contact. If you accidently touch the sores or fluids. Wash your hands! Thoroughly, to avoid spreading the infection. I repeat these cautions ad nauseum throughout this book. Wash your hand!

Question? Where do you live on "the boy in the bubble" Vetter Curve? At what levels of isolation, restriction, protection, and justification do you exist? Yes, it's possible to avoid being infected by the sexual predator. But it may not be worth the extreme "bubble" measures to eliminate the herpes risk. Think about it. Do you want to avoid touching other human beings? Abstain from all sexual contact: vaginal, oral, anal, or other? Doesn't sound appealing or possible. But you can reduce the chance of getting infected by being in a long-term, mutually monogamous relationship. With both partners having tested negative. It's important to understand that "nothing" fully protects against herpes 100%. It occurs in both men and women's oral cavities or genital areas that are not covered by contraceptives: the mouth and tongue, or anus, rectum, perineum, and testicles.

CAUTION: many who are infected with the herpes virus don't know it. They've never been tested or had an active outbreak. Even so, they're still capable of passing it on. (Below: 2016_11_10 Sacral Eczema Herpeticum)

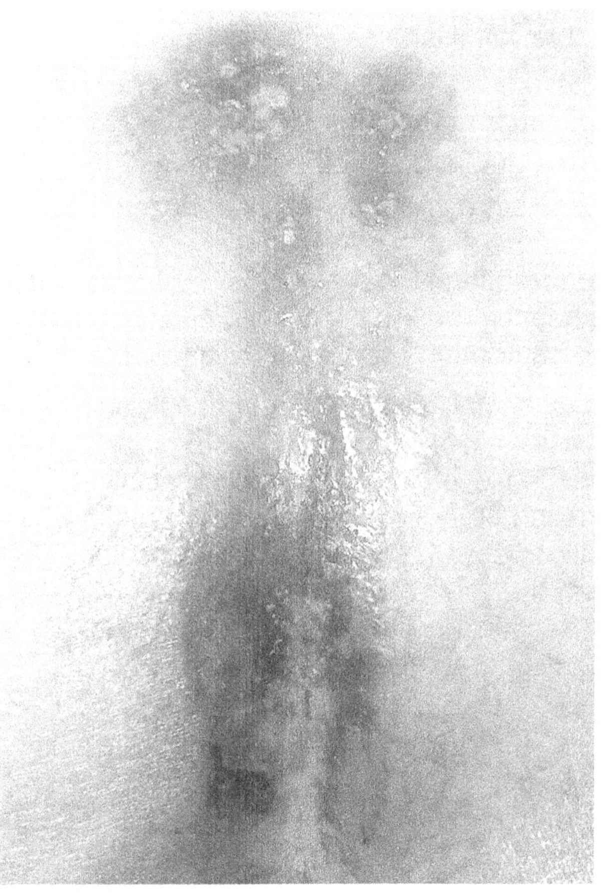

C. Eczema Challenges

The cause of Eczema, Atopic Dermatitis, is not fully understood. However, many times, hay fever and asthma are associated with it. Heredity seems to also play a part, since nearly 70% of eczema patients have at least one family member with either eczema, hay fever, or asthma. Food allergies are thought to be a causative factor, but this has not been proven. The prevailing thought in medicine, it's caused by an *abnormal allergic response* by the body's immune system. This may be short-sighted, since it's best to look at a person's entire lifestyle, including diet, environment, and their toxic load.

Since the skin is often called the "window of balance" of the body, it may be important to address the cause(s) rather than just treating topical symptoms. In many cases of eczema, the body seems to be trying to eliminate internal toxins.

According to Natural Medicine, causes of eczema include:

1. Food allergies from dairy products, eggs, grains (wheat), soy, and nuts.
2. A deficiency of Essential Fatty Acids (EFAs).
3. Damaged, clogged, or a toxic liver, kidneys, and/or lungs.
4. A vitamin and mineral deficiency.
5. A vitamin D deficiency.
6. A deficiency in Chloride of Potassium.
7. Overconsumption of table salt. Use *sea salt*.
8. Irritable Bowell Syndrome, constipation, disorders of the digestive tract.
9. Excess consumption of sugar and alcohol.
10. Chemicals that disturb the gut flora.
11. Poor digestion and toxins are a common cause of eczema sufferers.

CONSIDERATION: Do you frequently use antacids? Antacids reduce stomach acid. Contrary to TV commercials, you need more (not less) stomach acid to digest food properly. Poor digestion and associated complications can lead to skin problems.

Since the skin is the body's largest elimination organ (through sweating), it is a way for the body to rid itself of toxic waste, gases, and oils. These toxins, and nutritional deficiencies, may be the primary underlying cause of eczema. A clogged liver, malfunctioning kidneys, lung issues, as well as constipation, may increase toxins circulating through the blood, and being eliminated through the skin as eczema. Chronic skin conditions generally reflect the health of the digestive tract. Treating the liver, kidneys, and bowels with mild alternative remedies can positively affect eczema and an important part of any back-to-health protocol. eczema is usually expressed in three distinct stages defined by age of onset:

1. Infancy
2. Childhood
3. Adolescence/adulthood

More than half of all eczema cases will appear during the first year of life. A total of 45% of all eczema develops in **infants 2 to 6 months** of age with itching, redness, and small bumps on the cheeks, forehead or scalp that may later spread to the trunk. The **childhood** phase of eczema eruption commonly occurs between the **ages of 4 and 10 years**, and is characterized by raised, itchy, scaly bumps on the face and/or trunk also accompanied by dryness and thickening of the skin. The **adolescent/adult** phase appears at or **after the time of puberty** and is distinguished by itchy, dry, scaly skin that may continue into adulthood.

There is considerable evidence for *immune dysregulation* in individuals with eczema. Although there are still many unanswered questions, a pre-disposition is known to play a key role in eczema. The risk of childhood eczema is two to three times higher in children with a maternal or paternal history. Thank you Mom and Dad. **Hyperlink reference** may not be valid. http://bit.ly/2E9bZFp

Do You Have Eczema?

If you suspect that you have eczema (**Atopic Dermatitis**), ask yourself:

1. Is the rash itchy?
2. Is there dry skin with a red or scaly rash?
3. If the rash has occurred in the past, is the skin thicker in that area?

If you answered yes to any one of these questions, the next step is to consult your health care provider or a specialist that treats eczema patients. They will get an in-depth history and may perform additional diagnostic tests, including:

1. A detailed medical history,
2. Blood tests and skin biopsy, and
3. Allergy tests.

Medical History

A detailed medical history is probably the most important and reliable tool for diagnosing eczema. Your doctor will focus on when the rash appears, where it appears, and how often. They will also ask about itching and possible triggers, such as foods, allergens, temperature changes, and other aspects in your environment that create flare-ups.

Tests for Eczema

While a medical history is critical, additional tests can help support the eczema diagnosis.

Blood tests: One such test looks for high levels of a molecule called IgE antibody. Blood levels of these are elevated in people with atopic diseases, including eczema.

Skin biopsy: To rule out other skin diseases such as cancer or psoriasis. A pathologist then examines the skin sample under a microscope.

Allergy skin testing: to show sensitization or lack of sensitization to specific allergens.

Patch testing: In this test, small patches covered with allergenic chemicals are placed on the skin for 48 hours, then removed and the skin reaction is evaluated for possible allergies to fragrances, metals, lanolin, rubber, etc.

Buccal swabs: The inside of the cheek can be swabbed with a cotton applicator to get cells as a source of DNA material to look for mutations in the Filaggrin gene, one of the causes of eczema.

Allergy Challenge Tests

If your medical history points to atopic dermatitis, then your healthcare provider can move on to specific tests, known as "challenges," to determine if it's something in your environment or the food you eat that aggravates your condition. You can then try to avoid these specific triggers.

However, research suggests that genes are the determining causes of eczema and other atopic diseases. This means that you are more likely to have atopic dermatitis, food allergies, asthma and/or hay-fever if your parents or other family members have ever had eczema. Although there is no known way to keep from getting eczema, it may be possible to minimize the number of outbreaks by avoiding its triggers. These fall into four basic categories:

1. **Things that dry out your skin** is a key feature of eczema. If you live in an environment of low humidity or extreme air temperatures (either hot or cold), it can remove moisture from the skin. Harsh soaps and frequent washing without applying moisturizers can bring on flare-ups.

2 **Emotional stressors:** Anger, frustration, anxiety, and day to day stressors can cause the skin to flush and trigger eczema.

3. **Allergies:** Allergic reactions often trigger a rash and a general itchy feeling. Two types of allergens are commonly linked to symptoms: (1) Airborne allergens including dust mites, animal dander, and pollen, and (2) food triggers caused such as milk, eggs, peanuts, soy, wheat, and fish.

4. **Skin infections:** Bacterial and viral infections of the skin, like herpes, can bring on eczema flares. A common bacterial culprit is Staphylococcus Aureus ("staph"). The herpes viruses, which cause cold or genital sores, are also linked to flare-ups. In addition, outbreaks of herpetic lesions around the eyes should be of extra concern and be immediately evaluated by an eye specialist.

IMPORTANT: people with atopic dermatitis should consult with their doctor before getting vaccinated, especially the smallpox vaccine. Atopic dermatitis is a highly individual disease. Some patients are sensitive to many eczema triggers; others react to only one. It is important for you to identify your specific triggers.

Medications and Eczema Treatments

Steroid medicines that are applied to the skin are called *topical* steroids. Topical steroids fight inflammation. They are very helpful when a rash is not well controlled. They are available in many forms for the treatment of eczema, such as ointments, creams, lotions, gels and even tape. They are made from low to super potent strengths. Do not substitute one topical steroid for another without your healthcare provider's advice. Used correctly, **topical** steroids are safe and an effective treatment for atopic dermatitis. Be cautious with steroid **pills** or **liquids**, such as prednisone, because of side effects and the rash often comes back with a vengeance after they're stopped.

Topical Calcineurin Inhibitors (TCIs) are medicines that are applied to the skin for the treatment of eczema. They treat inflammation but are not steroids. TCIs don't cause steroid side effects. A common side effect of TCIs is skin burning, but generally does not last long. TCIs include Protopic® ointment (tacrolimus) and Elidel® cream.

Topical PDE4 Inhibitors (PDE4) are medicines applied to the skin to treat inflammation but are also not steroids. They are approved for children 2 years and older with mild to moderate atopic dermatitis. PDE4s include Eucrisa® (crisaborole). Skin and scalp products that contain coal-tar extracts have long been used to treat and reduce itching and rash. Tar shampoos, such as T-Gel®, are often helpful for red and itchy scalp. For scalp scaling or flaking, T-Sal® or Head and Shoulders® may be helpful.

Oral antihistamines are used to control allergy symptoms and can help reduce itching from atopic dermatitis. Some antihistamines cause drowsiness but can make you feel less itchy and help you sleep. eczema creams and lotions that contain antihistamines or anesthetics (for numbing) should be avoided. They can cause skin irritation and allergic skin reactions.

Phototherapy exposure to natural sunlight or ultraviolet light often helps people with atopic dermatitis. https://bit.ly/3nAhEvt

Psychological Counseling often helps people with eczema who often struggle with a poor self-image and low self-esteem. In severe cases, the appearance of their skin can invite teasing and, especially with children, interfere with peer relationships. https://bit.ly/3P6xeuF

Skin Infections caused by bacteria (e.g., impetigo), fungus (e.g., athlete's foot), but especially the herpes virus (either genital herpes or cold sores) can complicate eczema symptoms. A skin infection can quickly get out of control. Please, call your healthcare provider ASAP if you think you have an infection!

D. Isolation

Loneliness is a problem for many people, but especially for chronic herpes and eczema sufferers. What if we could enjoy loneliness? Change it from a negative, painful experience, to a positive one. Just as it's not the ingredients (being alone) in life, but how we relate to them that's important. So, it is with being alone. It's how our minds relates to being alone.

Our Herpeticum experience often lacks a sense of humor. I don't mean telling jokes, being funny, or criticizing other people and then laughing at them. They already do that enough to us. But having a light affect. Not beating our herpes and/or eczema experiences into the ground. Appreciating the reality of life for what it is. Weird and wonderful, fleeting, mysterious, almost humorous, almost dreamlike, and yet, it's not mocking us. With that realization we come to accept personal responsibility for uplifting our Herpeticum experience of loneliness.

Create more peace and harmony even if infected with eczema and herpes and live alone? Loneliness doesn't destroy happiness. It's our relationship with our disease and being alone that can create feelings of loneliness if we allow it.

If we break down the barricades of shame, guilt, and feelings of isolation that envelopes herpes and eczema, then the walls of feeling lonely crumble. The disease is now part of us. A teammate in our loneliness. It's nothing to be ashamed of. *"I have the life ingredient of eczema and/or herpes, that if not careful can transform into Herpeticum. I acknowledge that, and people still like me. Even more important, I like me."*

We get afraid of loneliness because of our self-identification with the disease. Then it's not a stretch to think of *ourselves* as the *disease*. Very often loneliness is an identity crisis. If we're constantly identifying with our disease, even when by ourselves, we can get confused about who we are.

We can't control the body with its illnesses, just as we can't control the ingredients of life, or our wives, husbands, and other people. When we stop trying to control people, places, and life itself, then life will stop disturbing us. The problem of loneliness is solved. It's amazing how still and blissful we get when we let go of control.

Spiritual Power, and not the false sense of control power, is the way to peace and happiness. It's in our relationship to *People, Places, and Things* wherein lies the problem and the solution.

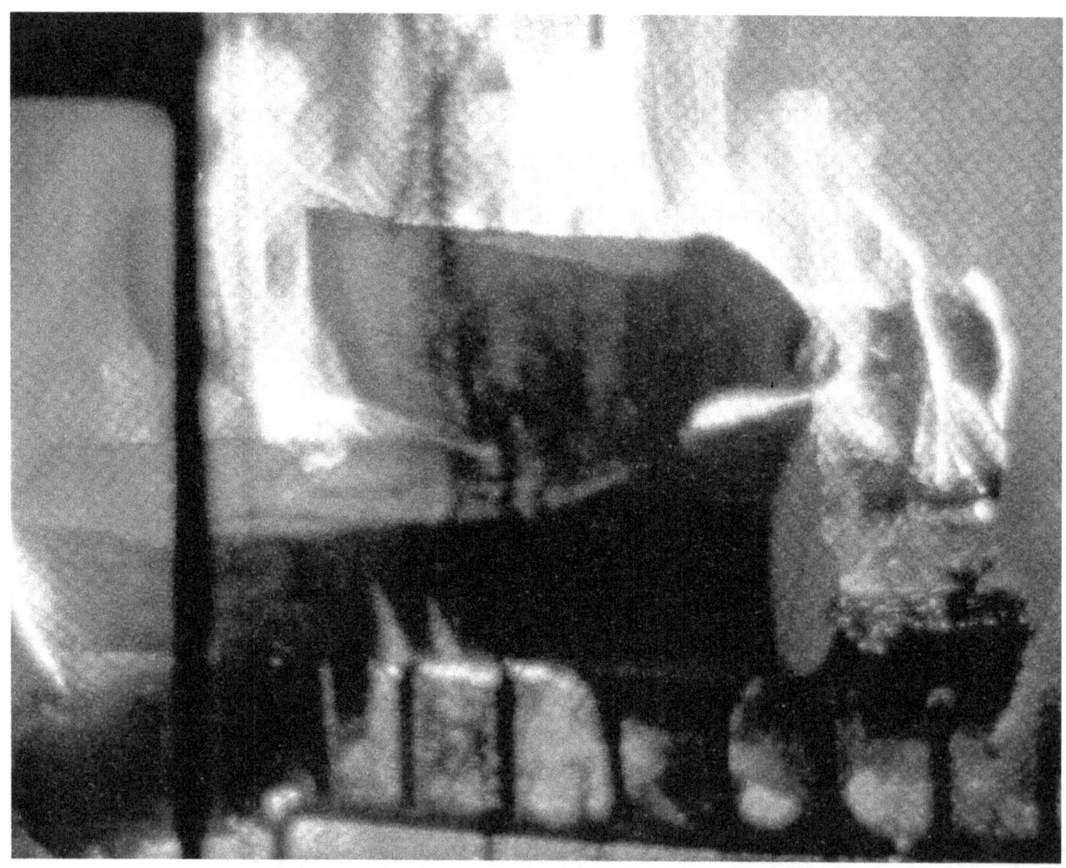

The Flames of Eczema Herpeticum

Chapter 4: Eczema Herpeticum

Herpes and Eczema are most often two separate diseases. Bothersome, but they seldom cause serious complications. Most herpes outbreaks and eczema flare-ups heal on their own without difficulties. With one grave exception: when an eczema flare-up, usually atopic dermatitis (AD), are infected with the herpes virus (HSV-1 or HSV-2). A chance encounter can develop into **Eczema Herpeticum (EH).** A rare, but serious, and even fatal infection if treatment is not properly initiated. Other viruses besides herpes may occasionally be responsible for Herpeticum, such as Coxsackievirus A16, the cause of hand foot and mouth disease https://bit.ly/3yDNuOm.

A herpes infection on an eczematous area of the skin can quickly spread into a painful, blistery, oozing rash, like an out-of-control brush fire. If left untreated, it can spread to vital organs throughout the body. On rare occasions it is still fatal. October 2016 Genital Herpes and eczema turned unpleasant for the author.

I started feeling unwell, with a slight fever and swollen lymph nodes in the groin area. In addition, the following symptoms appeared:

1. The blisters appeared similar to each other.
2. They were filled with a clear yellow fluid.
3. Blood-stained, red, purple, black in color.
4. New blisters had central dimples (umbilication).
5. They started to weep and/or bleed.
6. Older blisters crusted over and formed sores (erosions).
7. Most lesions healed over two-months.
8. White scars are still visible today.

Secondary bacterial infection with staphylococci or streptococci can lead to complications that includes impetigo and/or cellulitis. On rare occasion, acute Eczema Herpeticum may affect multiple organs, including the eyes, brain, lung, and liver, if not treated properly can still be fatal.

See Photograph Next Page
Author's Sacrum Infection with
Eczema Herpeticum, November 2016

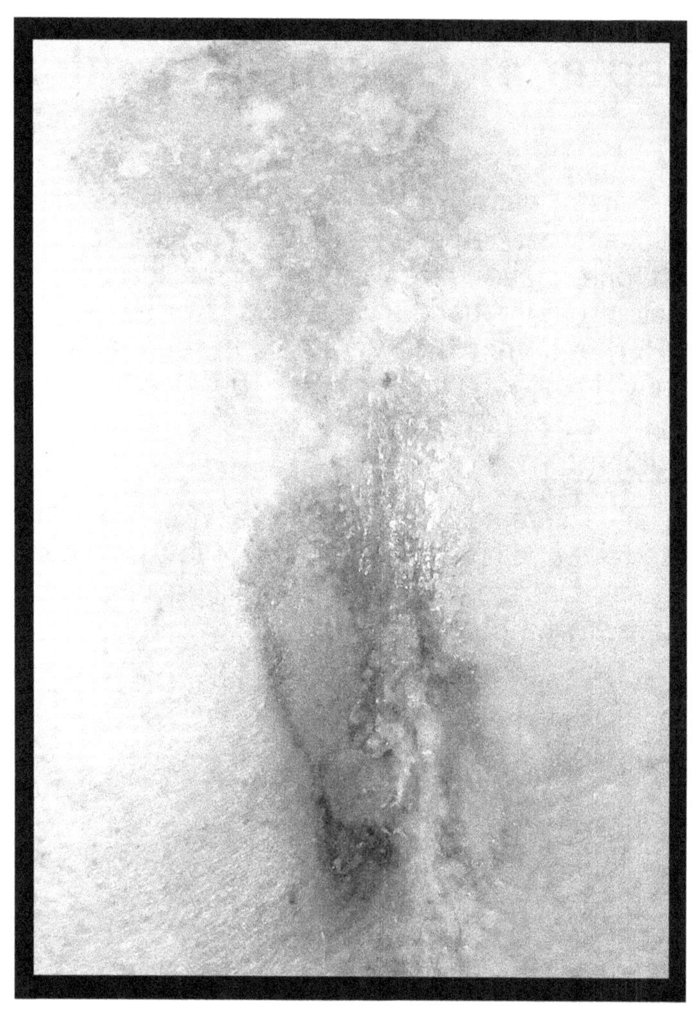

November 11, 2016, Eczema Herpeticum (EH)

Technically, Herpeticum is a form of *Kaposi Varicelliform Eruption* (KVE). A blistery rash that usually arises from atopic dermatitis (AD). Eczema Herpeticum can progress from a single rash/outbreak into an infection that quickly spreads throughout the body. http://bit.ly/2DJI35r It's important to be diagnosed early and treated promptly. The most common treatment is antiviral medication that varies in dose depending on the patient's immune status. To diagnose Eczema Herpeticum doctors swab the lesions and culture it.

"Just like other HSV infections, Eczema Herpeticum can recur. In an immune compromised patient, the mortality rate is reported to be as high as 6% to 10% and even 50%. Timely diagnosis and treatment of Eczema Herpeticum is important to avoid severe complications." http://bit.ly/2DJXdnl

Since Eczema Herpeticum is uncommon, it is sometimes misdiagnosed as impetigo. A detailed history makes a significant difference for an accurate diagnosis. Even though other viruses cause Herpeticum, it's most frequent with herpes infections. That's why it's referred to as **Eczema Herpeticum (EH).**

EH can require long-term preventative treatment. My outbreaks lasted from October 2016 to April 2017. I was prescribed Acyclovir and a topical anti-bacterial cream to be applied as necessary to any lesions. At first, I thought it was just a severe case of eczema. But as the rash and ulcers spread, my sacrum started to look like the endgame of a flame thrower. I knew something was amiss. Gratefully, so did my doctors. Even though nothing was cultured, they were pre-emptive.

After applying Rx ointments, I'd cover lesions with large non-stick sterile Band-Aids. EH's rash surrounded my sacrum and anus. Number "two" turned into a two-hour clean up. I was not hospitalized because I'm stubborn, but also took oral antiviral therapy for several weeks. Most advanced cases are hospitalized and put on intravenous treatment.

It's been almost 5 years since my last herpes or EH outbreak. The doctors warned me that long-term outcomes are inconsistent and recurrence rates high. I was to remain vigilant and prepared for regular therapy. Lesions and outbreaks healed slowly, and at times worsened until I started the Hermes Protocol. Although EH occurred on my sacrum with HSV-2, it's more often caused by Cold Sores (HSV-1) with eczema flare-ups on the face, neck, or upper trunk. Herpeticum symptoms do not appear right away. They typically show up a week or two after being infected with the herpes virus.

Eczema Herpeticum symptoms can include a blistery rash that appears in clusters and often covers a large area. The blister can break open, be itchy, painful, weep, bleed, and/or have pus-like yellow fluid inside. As the rash appears, it feels like the flu with swollen lymph nodes, fever, chills, and fatigue.

Herpeticum complications may involve:

1. **Long-term scarring** from slow healing blisters.

2. **Herpes infection** in the cornea of the eye, Herpetic Keratitis, can lead to blindness if left untreated.

3. **Prompt treatment is essential**. If herpes spreads to the brain, lungs, or liver, organ failure may occur. I'm not sure we want to live without our brain or liver or even without our lungs.

Herpeticum frequently occurs with these skin conditions:

1. Atopic Dermatitis (most often),
2. Seborrheic Dermatitis,
3. Irritant Contact Dermatitis,
4. Burns, and
5. Psoriasis.

EH's primary victims are infants and children. However, anyone with a compromised immune system is fair game and susceptible. With eczema, please avoid contact with anyone who has a Cold Sore or Genital Herpes. Those with partners may want to sleep in the guest room or couch. Wait until the abscess leaves the heart fonder. Do not share eating utensils, cosmetics, clothing, glassware, or any other item that touched active herpes lesions.

If you are in a Relationship:

1. Keep herpes infections under control.
2. Keep eczema flare-ups under control.
3. Keep both under control.
4. If you're active, avoid contact with others.
5. Move to North Dakota and live alone; and
6. Exaggerated and glib, but not farfetched.

Suggestions that may help:

Know your triggers. It may be easier to avoid eczema flare-ups than herpes outbreaks. Or it may not. Avoid both whenever possible. With an active eczema flare-up, ask your doctor whether it's a good idea to take antiviral meds until the eczema subsides. It may keep herpes from breaking out at the same time, in the same spot.

Avoid scratching your skin. It may cause cracks or breaks, leaving it vulnerable to infections. Coconut oil is both a moisturizer and protectant

.

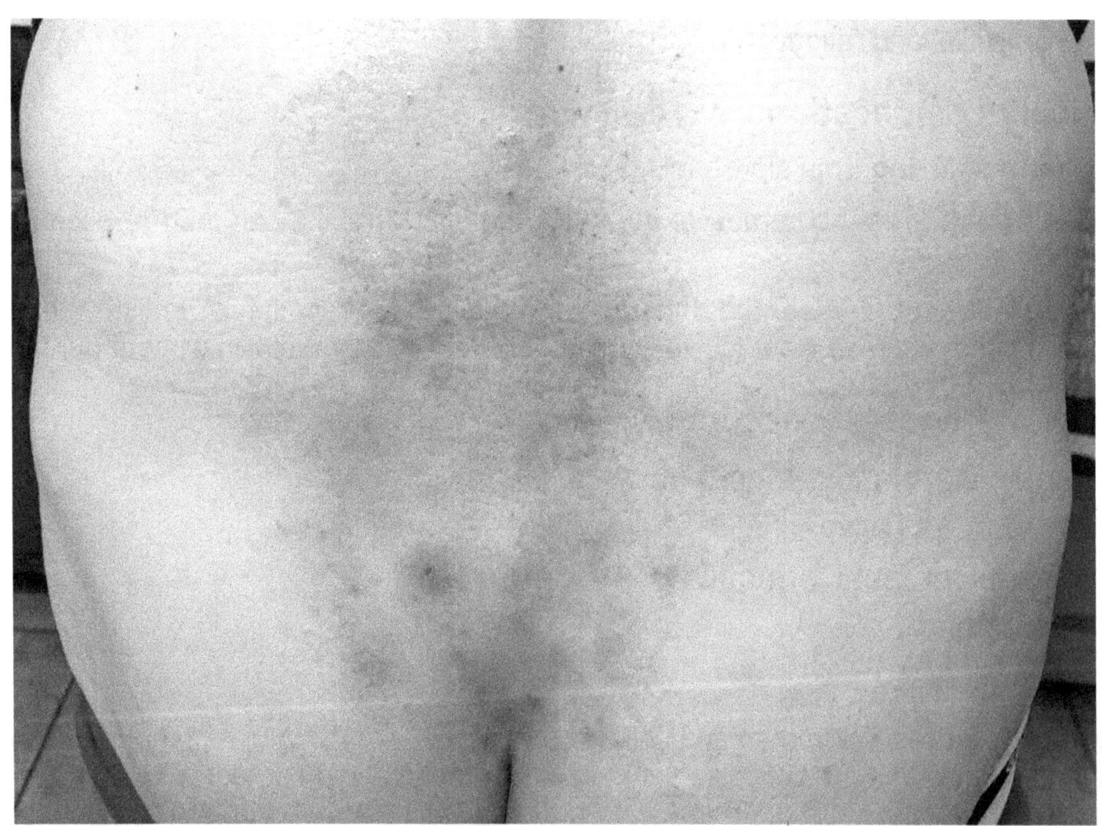

October 2016 Sacral Eczema Herpeticum Outbreak

Use herpes and/or eczema medications as prescribed. Both oral and topical creams can promote eczema healing, relieve itching and inflammation. With an active Genital Herpes outbreak, be careful. Creams that are beneficial for eczema may not be for herpes. eczema corticosteroid creams come in different strengths, from mild over the counter (OTC) treatments, to strong prescription medicines. For Genital Herpes, I used an MMS and DMSO solution several times a day to ameliorate and resolve symptoms (See Chapter 8, Chlorine Dioxide and DMSO).

Keep track of your herpes and eczema symptoms. *Always* see a doctor if they worsen! Especially if a fever is present. Protect affected skin with a non-stick Band-Aid, especially near the sacrum. Wash hands frequently and avoid direct contact with lesions whenever possible. Use a Q-Tip for medication ointments or creams.

Avoid sex with an active outbreak. No matter what, make sure to wear protections. A latex condom acts as a barrier against sexually transmitted infections, including herpes. But like anything else in life, except death and time, it's not a guarantee. Although our focus is Genital Herpes, the Hermes Protocol helped both herpes and eczema outbreaks. (Below: 2016 Sacral Eczema Herpeticum)

Chapter 5: Pillars of Health

Difficulties are part of life. It's my job not to magnify or empower them. If they start to overwhelm me, I know what to do. You will, too, by the time you finish this book.

For many years I was focused and determined to find a magic "silver-bullet." Like a court order, directing Genital Herpes to cease and desist. Stop! No more out-break activity. But I never found an appellate court to rescind or reverse my outbreak history.

After decades in herpes purgatory, today I'm outbreak free for almost 5 years. Healing and remission occurred through the Hermes Protocol and in the four pillars of health. The goal is to stretch beyond the physical line of attack. To incorporate the mental, emotional, and spiritual realms because they have a greater influence on our physical health than we give them credit.

Four Pillars of Health:

1. **Physical**
2. **Emotional**
3. **Mental**
4. **Spiritual**

The pillars of health are united in the Hermes Protocol through nutrition, diet, lifestyle, supplementation, mindfulness practices, detoxification, and alternative protocols. Given the right conditions, the body will maintain in a state of dynamic equilibrium called "good-health" or "well-being." The remainder of this book will address the four pillars of health and how they counter the effects of the three adversaries to health.

Three Adversaries to Health

1. **Deficiency**
2. **Toxicity**
3. **An Uncontrolled Mind**

The Hermes Protocol offers a variety of supplements and protocols to support the body's recovery from deficiency, toxicity, and an uncontrolled mind.

A. Undervalued Pillars

Beside the Physical aspect of health, there are the Mental, Emotional, and Spiritual components. All intricately interrelated.

Mental: the ability to think through problems logically.

Emotional: the ability to feel what others are experiencing.

Spiritual: our soul, which is beyond thought and the mind.

One option, when faced with not knowing the cause of a challenging and complicated illness like Herpeticum, is to "change" our perception of the problem. That's often difficult. When we live by *"what-you-see-is-what-there-is,"* then physical reality is what you get. Life loses its charm and insightful emotional and spiritual component. It can still be valid and an "efficient" way to live, but Spirit is "missing." We all know the "by-the-numbers" type. They only follow the instructions mentality. There is a 'dead-zone' or detached feeling. As we all know from our dating experience, *"Looks can deceive: that's why perception and reality don't always match up."* Be mindful! The visual-physical-ego loves to trick and treat.

Mental

Even though a healthy diet is vital, it's like sitting on a one-legged stool. It works for circus performers and acrobatic chefs. There is no magic or *"Hi-Ho Silver Bullet, eczema, and herpes… away!"* Everybody's support system needs to harmonize to protect the body from infections. The body-mind connection is one more example of that.

While the expression "It's all in your head" may refer to one's mental state, it doesn't diminish the physical symptoms that can arise from mental or emotional distress. People seem more willing to accept the mind/body connection to back pain than they are to eczema or herpes. That said, there is little dispute that stress is detrimental to both.

Not all the news about herpes infections and the mind is benign. *"Persistent herpes infections may be associated with cognitive impairments,"* reports *Psychological Medicine.* Researchers have found herpes virus infections cause cognitive impairment during and after acute encephalitis. Herpes Simplex Encephalitis (HSE) is a viral infection of the central nervous system. Fifty percent of its victims are over 50 years of age. http://bit.ly/2Gqd9wl

University of Michigan study, links HSV-1 to mental impairment throughout life. *"This study is a first step in establishing an association between these viruses and cognition across a range of ages in the U.S. population."* http://bit.ly/2rHykqE

These findings present a potential future mental health crisis. More than one third of the U.S. population tests positive for the herpes virus by early childhood. Although most individuals are not symptomatic, *"If HSV-1 begins to have impact on cognitive function early in life, HSV-1 infection in childhood may have important consequences for educational attainment and social mobility across the lifespan."* Something to think about. Since many assume, they're fortunate to only have Cold Sores and not genital sores.

Emotional

According to Dr. Mercola and the *Journal of Neuroanatomy*, microwave radiation from cell phones, Wi-Fi routers, and computers is associated with many neuropsychiatric disorders. http://bit.ly/2EhRupV

"Depression is anger turned inward, and a Limbic-cortical dysregulation, and monoamine imbalance." In plain English. Please, be careful with your iPhone. Try not hold it near your head. Anyone struggling with emotional issues related to anxiety or depression, limit your exposure to wireless technology. Turn Wi-Fi off at night and try not to carry your cellphone on your body. At home, keep portable home phones, cellphones, and other electric devices out of your bedroom. At the very "most" a long distance from your bed.

In 2017, suicide rates were at a 30-year high. Mental disorders the second most common cause of disability. Prescription drug abuse and overdose deaths a public health emergency. Opioid pain killers are among the most lethal, psychiatric drugs. In 2013, anti-anxiety benzodiazepine accounted for nearly one-third of prescription overdose deaths. Emotions can kill you, directly and indirectly.

Four "emotional" tactics to speed up the process of adjusting to herpes outbreaks and/or eczema rashes:

1. **First,** it's normal to be emotionally stressed with herpes infections and eczema rashes. Give yourself time to adjust, and remember, it will get easier.

2. **Second,** understand that herpes is like most infections. They can be managed.

3. **Third,** if feeling emotionally isolated, find an internet support group. Someone that will listen, even if counseling is the only option. To start, call a close friend or the National STI Hotline 1-800-232-4636 to speak to a counselor. There are many online support groups, or in person group sessions, that can help you cope. http://bit.ly/2DH8jJD

4. **Fourth,** do not assume anything. Herpes is often more mental than physical. It will not prevent anyone from being involved in a long-term relationship. There are millions, millions, and millions of couples all over the world who deal with Genital Herpes every day, and they make it work. Remember, you're not alone.

Six steps to managing stress better:

1. **Get enough sleep.** The more rested, the better at handling stress.
2. **Balance your diet.** Eat plenty of veggies and limit sugary foods.
3. **Exercise** in moderation relieves stress.
4. **Reach out.** Being with people and having fun can help.
5. **Relax.** Be content.
6. **Yoga, EFT, and meditation** are all soothing and healing.

Although persistent stress may lead to outbreaks and flare-ups, the daily little annoyances we face are not stressful enough to trigger herpes or eczema symptoms. However, there is one stress factor that can knock down the front door to your peace of mind. It can also be more hazardous to your health than smoking or obesity. It's called loneliness. The Hermes Protocol addresses those feelings in detail. Here's what Dr. Mercola had to say about it.

"An estimated 42.6 million Americans over the age of 45 suffer from chronic loneliness, and more than 25 percent of the U.S. population lives alone."

"Loneliness is associated with higher blood pressure and higher risk of heart disease, stroke, dementia, depression and lower survival rates for breast cancer patients."

"Loneliness is more hazardous to your health than obesity, raising your risk of early death by as much as 50 percent."

Thake-home message: don't isolate because of Herpeticum. It can be more consequential and damaging than the rashes themselves.

According to the American Osteopathic Association, which commissioned the Harris Poll cited above, loneliness plays a role in many chronic health conditions. These include pain, drug or alcohol abuse, depression, increased risk for Alzheimer's disease, heart attacks, stroke, and lower survival rates for breast cancer patients. And if that wasn't enough, people who are lonely are more likely to experience:

1. **Higher levels of stress,** more Herpeticum rashes.
2. **Poor sleep** for more herpes outbreaks.
3. **Increased inflammation**, more eczema flare-ups.
4. **Reduced immune function**, more outbreaks, flare-ups, rashes.

Emotional-Physical Connection

It's truly overwhelming how our emotions can influence overall health. A powerful force that either bolsters or undermines the immune system and our well-being. Epigenetics believes environmental factors such as stress and diet directly influence our genetic expression. It is the expression of our genes, not the genes themselves that determines whether we develop certain diseases or age prematurely. Guess where the herpes virus hides out? You guessed it. In our genetic DNA.

If you are chronically lonely and in a state of persistent herpes outbreaks or eczema flare-ups, our negative "emotions" will influence the expression of our genes and affect the risk of developing even more diseases. Don't isolate. With or without an active lesion, flare-up, or infections. Live as if you are the most beloved child of a Divine Universe. Here are some suggestions and strategies that can help overcome the struggles with loneliness and isolation:

1. **Join a club.** Meetup.com is a source of local clubs and get-togethers.

2. **Learn a new skill.** Enroll in a class or take an educational course.

3. **Consider a digital cleanse.** If Social Media has overtaken your life, consider taking a sabbatical. Take steps to meet "real" people in person. Recent research shows Facebook may be more harmful than helpful to emotional well-being.

4. **Make effective use of digital media.** For some, a phone call or text is a much-needed lifeline. Examples of this include sending encouraging text messages to people who are experiencing outbreaks and struggling with loneliness.

5. **Exercise with others.** Joining a gym or a fitness directed club can open opportunities to meet like-minded people while improving physical fitness at the same time.

6. **Do local coffee shops** and farmers markets to develop a sense of community.

7. **Volunteer** to increase social interactions.

8. **Adopt a companion dog or cat** that can provide unconditional love and comfort. Studies show that owning a pet can help protect against loneliness, depression, and anxiety. https://www.petfinder.com is an excellent resource.

9. **As a last option, move and/or change jobs**. It's not the answer for everyone, but for some it may be worthwhile. Especially if it brings you closer to longtime friends or family.

Then relax, take it easy, and be content. Oh, one last thought and comment about the following platforms: Facebook, YouTube, Twitter, Instagram, Snapchat, Reddit, Pinterest, and LinkedIn. Take a break. As in, *"Time-Out."*

Like all addictions, momentary pleasures have a long-term dark side. Researchers found *"that people who used social media for more than 2 hours per day were twice as likely to feel socially isolated."* http://bit.ly/2GsMMX4 And that's not its most detrimental effect. The body is being poisoned by constant WIFI radiation, compromising the immune system, and intensifying Herpeticum rashes.

Spiritual

"There's a Spiritual Solution to Every Problem" is a book by Wayne Dyer that sums up what is often a neglected or forgotten pillar in Western Medicine, the spiritual aspect of health. http://amzn.to/2BBVJcJ

When confronted with a physical problem like Herpeticum we often depend on our mind's intellect to solve our health concerns and/or relationship difficulties. In Wayne Dyer's book, he shows us that there is a more powerful spiritual force at our fingertips that contains the solution to most problems by learning how to *"...unplug from the material world and awaken to the divine within."* To paraphrase Wayne Dyer, *"The mind (thinking) is the source of problems. Your heart (Spirit) holds the answers to solving them."* The book begins with these words *"You have been looking the wrong way."*

B. Your Immune System

Most miracle products work marginally or not at all. They address the body's dashboard "Herpes" warning lights, which tells us there is a problem with the immune system. Taking the approach by fixing your warning lights, whether Genital Herpes or General Motors, is treating the symptom, not the cause.

Filling a deflated tire with air that has a nail-hole won't get you far. Yes, we can suppress symptoms by turning off the dashboard warning lights. But it won't fix the flat. In fact, other more serious side effects may surface if we continue to drive with a flat, or worse, on the rim. Then we'd be forced to treat those symptoms. And on, and on, and on, ad-infinitum. Until you finally abandon the clunker on some desolate highway.

Look under the hood. Go deeper into the immune system, and the warning lights will go off by themselves. Regrettably, many people just want a pill or quick fix to treat their symptoms. I don't blame them. I was one myself. Being healthy in today's toxic environment is a conscious, and often difficult, decision. But it's a responsibility we accept to be Herpes Free.

Five Immune Warning Signs:

1. Constantly Tired

Sometimes the car won't start in the morning. We need a push or a jump to get us going. This is a 21st Century epidemic. There are many potential causes for fatigue, some more innocuous than others. But when we're constantly tired, it may be time to see Dr. Feelgood.

2. Frequent Infections

The car seems to be running hot. At least that's what the manual said about the coolant light flickering on and off. But the mechanic said everything checked out OK. He thinks it might be a loose fuse or wiring in the dashboard. But while driving to work during a minor heat wave, steam is coming out from under the hood. So, you pull over and call Triple Health.

Dr. Feelgood says it might be your hormones, and that's why you can't cool down after a treadmill walk. It could also be the reason for frequent Cold Sore, urinary tract and yeast infections, red inflamed gums, persistent indigestion, and constipation. All potential warning signs of a compromised immune system.

3. Constantly Sick

Accidents happen. You hit a shopping cart in Costco's parking lot, or back into a pole at work. Everyone gets into accidents or gets sick occasionally. But if you're catching every cold or flu that says "Hello," it may be a sign that your immune system is compromised. You may need a tune-up and some lab work to make sure everything is OK.

4. Severe Allergies

As we age, our bodies, like automobiles, tend to rust more. Particularly if we live in an area of high humidity and severe winters. Then breaking out in rust is not that unusual. Allergies can also be a normal response. The same watery eyes during pollen season is probably nothing to worry about. But new and severe allergies may be an early warning sign that the immune system is malfunctioning. http://bit.ly/2GrkEne

5. Too Long to Heal

Did you notice the newly repainted driver's side door is starting to rust again? Like the time you cut yourself and it turned into a "Colloidal-Silver" emergency. It took forever to scab and heal? A compromised immune system can lead to significant delays in the healing process even for minor injuries. http://bit.ly/2GsVaFN

Keep in mind, these are only clues for immune complications. They can also happen for other reasons. The more informed we are as our own health advocates, the quicker Dr. Feelgood will be able to figure out what's wrong.

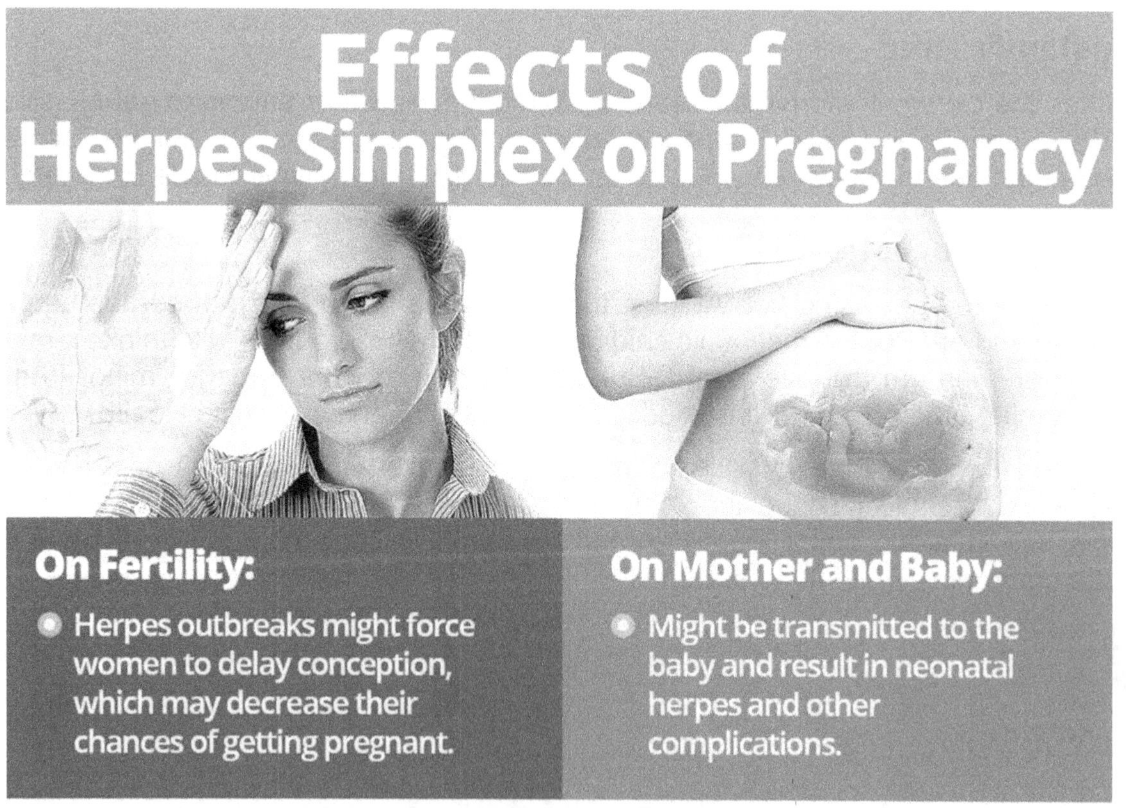

C. Hormones and Herpes

Hormones affect every pillar of "life," including the immune system and frequency of herpes outbreaks. Women can attest to that more so than men. Genital Herpes often coincides with their "cycle." Bloating, irritable mood, pelvic pain, or pressure are all common signs that a monthly period is coming soon. And for many women, this monthly guest often brings unwanted company, Genital Herpes.

Menses

To add offense to outbreaks, studies have confirmed that a women's menstrual period is one of the most common triggers for herpes outbreak. Stress the most common. For some women, outbreaks start as a burning or tingling sensation. A numbness or pain in the genital area, vagina, vulva, or buttocks. Others experience swollen lymph nodes, fever, chills, and headaches. They may also feel pain or burning in one leg, the bottom of their foot.

Antivirals can almost always shorten an outbreak with early recognition and treatment. While menses can trigger herpes outbreaks, the opposite is not true. Menstrual periods do not change with herpes infections. Sometimes women have the misperception that their menstrual irregularities are related to Genital Herpes outbreaks. That is questionable. If you have an active outbreak and missed your period, or it's changed in some way, talk to your doctor. It's probably not related to herpes. Remember, association is not always the cause.

Your Thyroid

Several scientific studies, http://bit.ly/2DYSMZn, "The Effects of Thyroid Hormone on HSV-1" suggest that *"hormone imbalances may cause virus reactivation."*

Do you want your health back? Are you ready to disable herpes infections? Regain lost energy and feel like a new self again? Then ask yourself, *"How important is my thyroid to my overall well-being and herpes outbreaks?* In one word. Critical, indispensable, serious, key, vital, significant. Oops! I didn't have time to list them "one" at-a-time.

Without a proper functioning thyroid, forget about it. When the thyroid is not performing well, neither are you. It can create havoc in people's lives. Together with the adrenals, it's responsible for making energy.

The thyroid controls virtually every cell, tissue, and organ in the body. If it produces too much hormone, it's called **hyper**thyroidism. The body's systems speed up. If it produces to little thyroid, they slow down--**hypo**thyroidism,

Untreated thyroid disease leads to a myriad of conditions and diseases. Including heart disease, osteoporosis, infertility, and yes, "herpes reactivation." Research shows that there is also a strong genetic link between thyroid disease and autoimmune diseases, including diabetes, arthritis, and anemia. Up to 60 percent of those with thyroid disease are unaware of their condition. Have your thyroid hormones checked by a health care specialist if you're cold when everyone else is warm. T*o find a good thyroid doc go to:*

https://stopthethyroidmadness.com/

Your Adrenals

If the thyroid is the conductor for well-being, the adrenals are the orchestra. Both need to be reading from the same sheet music and playing in harmony. Otherwise, the composition, like the music of our health, will clatter, crunch, and tinkle. Frequent overlooked causes of adrenal fatigue are chronic respiratory illnesses, and yes, herpes infections. It predisposes people to other chronic infections and respiratory problems.

Adrenal Fatigue symptoms include:

1. Autoimmune conditions
2. Chronic fatigue (always feeling tired)
3. Brain fog
4. Hormone imbalance
5. Insulin resistance
6. Lightheadedness
7. Decreased sex drive/libido
8. Moodiness and irritability
9. Depression
10. Muscle or bone loss
11. Skin ailments
12. Sleep disturbances
13. Weight gain
14. Sweet and salty food cravings.

Adrenal fatigue can occur after just one serious infection. Poorly performed dental procedures, such as a root canal, can also be a trigger. The more severe an infection, the more frequently it occurs, the longer it lasts, the more likely the adrenals are involved.

Prolonged or recurrent herpes infections gradually weaken the adrenals and the body's immune system, making it even more difficult to fight off herpes infections. Other infectious agents, such as parasites and fungus are also common triggers. It's not a surprise that adrenal fatigue and excessive tiredness are commonly associated with frequent herpes infections, including slower than normal healing. Immune weakness from waning adrenals can set the stage for *fibromyalgia*, for even greater debilitation. If there is a longer than normal recovery period, decreased stamina, and unwarranted tiredness after an illness or infection, look toward the adrenals.

Remember, stress triggers herpes outbreaks. Adequate adrenal support, a proper diet, healthy lifestyle, and effective stress management are crucial factors in minimizing stress-related herpes outbreaks.

Chapter 6: Start Today

Start today to improve your health. Some of these solutions are simple and may surprise you. For example:

1. **Eliminate** chlorinated faucet water.
2. **Drink** only natural, clean spring water.
3. **Add minerals** back into your diet.
4. **In the form** of natural sea salt or rock salt.
5. **Try** www.celticseasalt.com.

"The current IOM water recommendation *for men 19 years and older is drinking 3.7 liters (not quite a gallon) of pure, spring water per day (2.7 liters or almost 3 quarts for women)* *http://bit.ly/2BBeEEG* *This is your overall fluid intake per day, including anything you eat or drink containing water such as fruits or vegetables. You may need to drink more if you live in a hot climate, exercise often, have a fever, diarrhea, or vomiting."*

A top priority is putting trace minerals back into our bodies. Our soil is so depleted that we receive a fraction of the nutritional value from just a few years ago. To know the body's existing vitamin and mineral levels, and for appropriate supplementation, it is recommended that you do a **Hair Tissue Mineral Analysis (HTMA).** HTMA tests can be ordered through Trace Elements, Inc., or Analytical Research Labs, Inc. Both dependable and accurate Labs. **HTMA kits** can also be ordered through Robert Thompson, M.D., 907-260-6914, who uses Trace Elements, Inc. **Lawrence Wilson, M.D.,** at www.DrLWilson.com who uses Analytical Research Labs, Inc. Although Dr. Wilson no longer consults personally he has a list of approved "helpers" to initiate his program.

Dr. Charles Northern, a past leading scientist and researcher said, *"It's not commonly realized, however, that vitamins control the body's appropriation of minerals, and in the absence of minerals they have no function to perform. Lacking vitamins, the system can make some use of minerals, but lacking minerals, vitamins are useless."* Decades later, Dr. Linus Pauling, winner of two Nobel prizes, said, *"You can trace every sickness, every disease and every ailment to a mineral deficiency."* Clearly their warnings have fallen on minerally depleted ears.

A. Forks and Knives

Now that you've started your engine, let's take a lap around the track. Then eat. Diet plays an important part in any therapy or protocol, including the Hermes Protocol and Eczema Herpeticum. What's the old English proverb, *"Don't dig your grave with your own knife and fork."* But many of us do. *"I find that everyone is mineral-starved today, thanks to modern agricultural practices, stress and eating refined foods. Eating piles of cooked vegetables is the only way I know to obtain the nutrients everyone needs."* Dr. Lawrence Wilson

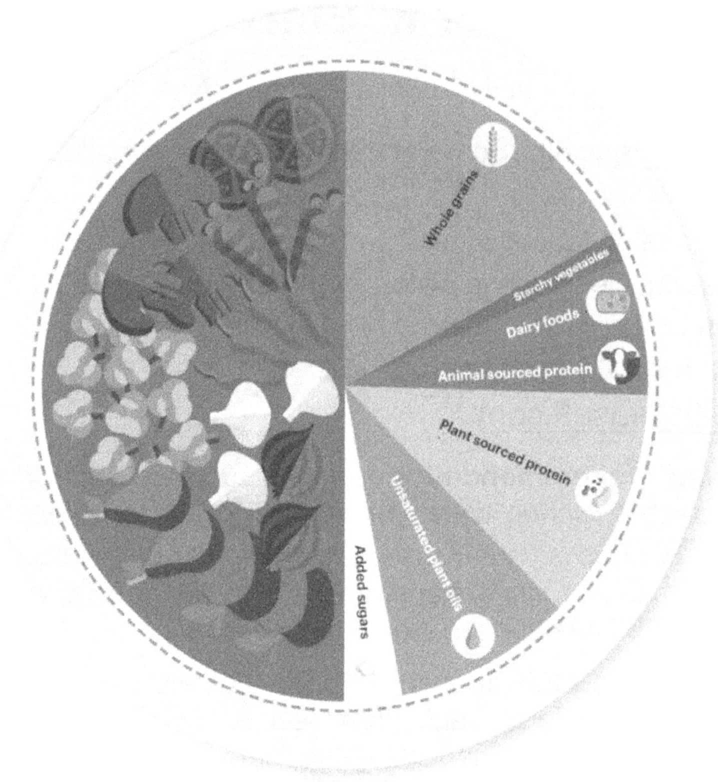

The "Diet" is restrictive, and not easy. Do your best. Remember the goal is to enhance the immune system to where it can keep herpes locked-up, and Eczema Herpeticum at bay

Not only are most people mineral-starved, but their digestion is also weak. What we're not missing from our diets are chemicals. There are over 3,000 chemicals permitted in food. Many damage or undermine our digestion and health. Organically grown food is best. Food from fast-food-restaurants is of poor quality and should be avoided.

Food over medicine and eating a plant-based diet is key in reclaiming good health. Plenty of "cooked" vegetables (not raw) with some animal protein each day.

Avoid all wheat, most fruits, and sugar. Keep meals simple. No more than two types—and if you include desert—three types of foods from proteins, carbs, and fats.

B. Healthy Food Choices

Focus on making healthy food and beverage choices to get the nutrients you need. Carbohydrates, protein, and fats are the three food groups that provide energy-producing nutrients. They can be broken down into: Grains, Vegetables, Fruits, Protein, Dairy, Oils, Solid Fats, and Added Sugars.

Recommendations to consider:

1. Eat plenty of cooked vegetables.
2. But not vegan or vegetarian.
3. Eat some animal protein daily.
4. For the first month avoid most fruit.
5. Instead, eat a few ounces of organic berries.
6. Keep meals to two groups (Carbs, Protein, and/or Fat).
7. Portion size varies according to age, height, lifestyle.
8. Eat slow and chew food thoroughly.
9. Do not eat the same foods each day.
10. Try eating only natural, whole foods.
11. In the beginning no powdered smoothies, or food bars.
12. Avoid drinking water with meals (some exceptions apply).
13. Organic food is best.
14. Avoid fast-food restaurants if possible.
15. Shun all refined flour, junk food, imitation, or chemicalized food.

What's wrong with eating fruit?

1. High in sugar, upsets the body's blood sugar.
2. Contains acids that can upset digestion.
3. Favors the growth of candida & other fungi.
4. Often sprayed with pesticides even when labeled organic.
5. Absorbs toxic potassium from N-P-K fertilizers.

Beverages: drink water. Buying spring water in 1 or 5-gallon jugs is fine. If you filter water, a carbon filter is adequate. Avoid reverse osmosis water. It lacks mineral content and is suspect of picking up plastic residue.

Alcoholic Beverages: a glass of snooty wine for all the wannabes? Say no. It's one of the most contaminated alcoholic beverages anywhere. Polluted with arsenic, even if labeled organic. Let me speak plainly, alcohol is bad for your health, even in moderation. Until recently, science-backed wisdom said alcohol in moderation was good for our health. New scientific research says that there is no safe alcohol limit. It's linked to more than 60 different diseases, with one drink a day increasing the risk of breast cancer by 4%. Even though "Responsible Drinking" is a 21st-century mantra, when it comes to cancer no amount of alcohol is safe.

Sugary Beverages: Just say "NO" to all sugary drinks. That includes all sodas, diet sodas, Kool-Aid, Gatorade, Recharge, and most energy drinks.

C. Nutrition for Herpes

The Do's: a diet high in Lysine helps control herpes outbreaks. Lysine is an amino acid that also strengthens the immune system to fight the virus.

Lysine-rich foods to consider:

1. **Fermented foods** like sauerkraut, miso, kefir, organic yogurt (in moderation).

2. **Add sea salt to meals** after cooking. They contain necessary source of minerals.

3. **Broccoli, Brussel sprouts** and cauliflower are our "best" friends for herpes.

4. **Chicken, beef, lamb, and sardines** are rich in Lysine. (Go light on the meat.)

5. **Homemade yogurt is rich in Lysine** and probiotics. A daily serving of yogurt supports the herpes healing process. Commercial products often contain gelatin or corn syrup that is high Arginine, which can cause more outbreaks.

6. **Drinking plenty of water improves** the alkaline balance of the body. Avoid caffeinated drinks, as caffeine increases Arginine levels.

7. **Coconut oil is an excellent source** of medium chain triglycerides. Its lauric and caprylic acid have antiviral effects.

The Don'ts: Arginine promotes the growth and replication of herpes. Eating Arginine rich foods may be OK on the condition the Arginine-Lysine ratio is in favor of Lysine. However, to be on the safe side of outbreaks, **limit the following high-Arginine foods:**

1. Seeds and nuts, and no Coconuts.
2. Coconut oil is fine, because it has few if any amino acids.
3. Orange juice
4. Chocolate
5. Any wheat products or Oats
6. Lentils
7. Protein supplements
8. Gelatin
9. Citrulline found in Watermelons, cantaloupes, and cucumbers.

Avoid most acidic foods and drinks below; they weaken the immune system:

1. Alcohol
2. Caffeine
3. All junk food
4. Eating too much red meat
5. All processed/white flour products
6. Food additives
7. Artificial sweeteners

D. Hacking the Mind

"Processed food is addictive *and promotes depression and early death."* That's according to Dr. Robert Lustig and his new book, *The Hacking of the American Mind: The Science Behind the Corporate Takeover of Our Bodies and Brains.*

Dr. Mercola interviewed Dr. Lustig http://bit.ly/2DYimxy about *"how food companies and government policy deceived the American public and turned food into a weapon of self-destruction."* And a herpes epidemic (author's hack), and a Herpeticum nightmare. According to Dr. Lustig, *"Sugar, processed foods, and other addictive substances, as well as chronic use of social media, releases dopamine that fuels addiction and depletes serotonin, which fuels depression, and will prematurely kill you."* But not before you have an endless string of herpes outbreaks, eczema flare-ups, Herpeticum complications, and think about packing it in, before you go on vacation.

In his book Dr. Lustig talks about, *"if you want to be happy, raise your serotonin levels, not dopamine (pleasure). There are four ways to increase serotonin, and all are free."*

1. **Making human connections.**
2. **Contributing to a larger cause.**
3. **Coping with stress (exercise and sleep).**
4. **Cooking real food.**

"Eating real food *that you prepare yourself is super important."* He emphasized the need for omega-3 fatty acids, especially DHA, a component of every cell in the body. More than 90% percent of the omega-3 fat in brain tissue is DHA.

As it turns out, Facebook does not count as a 'human' connection. Oh my gosh, what's my X going to do? *Social media generates dopamine, associated with pleasure. It drives addiction, not tryptophan and happiness. As dopamine goes up, serotonin and peace are flushed out. Online tweeting, texting, posting, surfing, and e-mailing is a major sponsor for momentary pleasure but long-term misery.*

Foods That Don't Work

Unfermented soy: blocks the uptake of iodine to the thyroid, starving it of an essential nutrient. This means no tofu, no soy milk, no edamame, and no soybean oil. Check labels. Soybean oil is cheap and in limitless products.

Gluten: avoid it. Period. It is mostly found in wheat, but also in other grains, including rye, barley, oats and spelt. Yes, oats, no matter what anyone says. Gluten is acidic, genetically modified, overproduced, and full of empty calories. U.S. wheat contains three times the gluten than European or South American wheat. It can also cause immune antibody production in the thyroid.

Sugar: like its evil twin tobacco, tricked consumers into believing it isn't as bad as it is. In January 2014, Eric Lawson was the fifth "Marlboro Man" to ride the non-addictive tobacco train into an early grave. His death was linked to smoking. So, what's the point? *Sugar* is the new *tobacco.*

Sugar Consumption per person past 300 + Years:

In 1700, consumed 4 pounds of sugar per year.

In 1800, increased to 18 pounds per year.

In 1900, consumption rose to 90 pounds.

In 2009, over 50% of Americans consumed 180 lbs of sugar per year.

Afterthought: I eat very little sugar. At most a few pounds a year. That means somebody out there is eating 360 pounds a year, or a pound of sugar a day! While shopping at Wegman's the other day, I checked out what a pound of sugar looks and feels like. I got goosebumps. Either that, or my candida or the herpes clan anticipated a Foie-Gras-Love-Fest.

If you're eating a half a pound of sugar a day, like the average American, please stop. It may be all the immune system needs to be on the road to recovery and end Genital Herpes outbreaks.

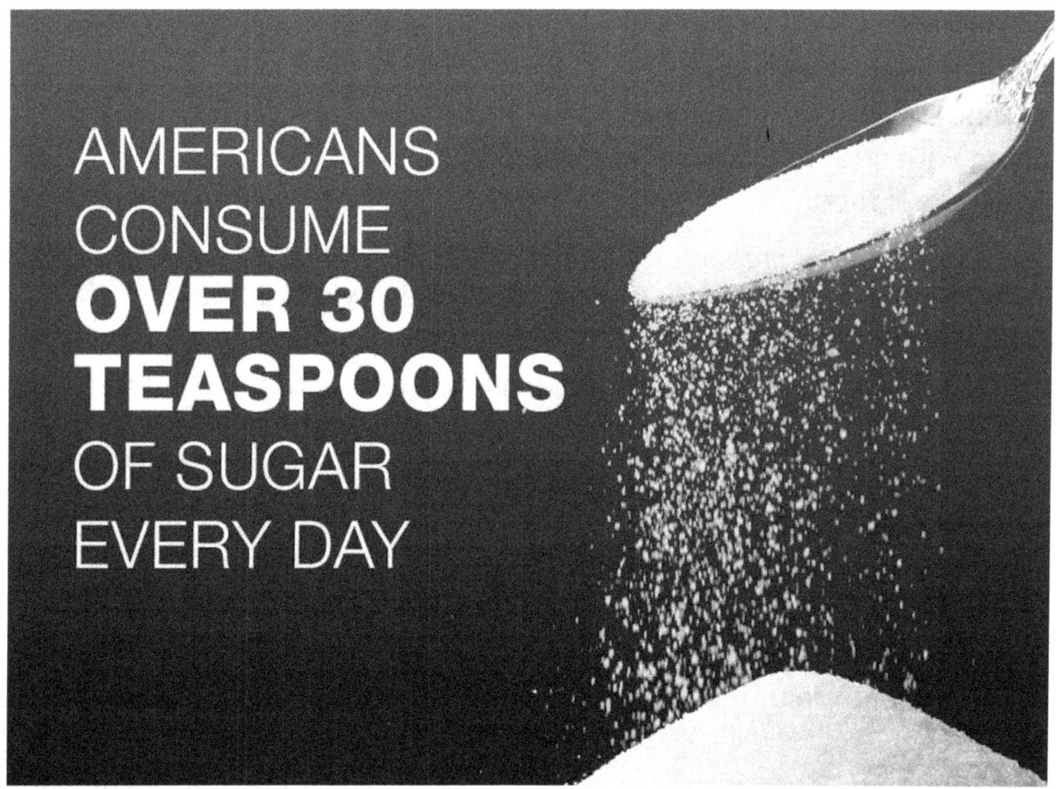

Chapter 7: Lifestyle Influences

According to Barbara Fredrickson, https://bit.ly/3bRHRD4 a psychologist and positive-emotions researcher, *"Most Americans have two positive experiences for every negative one."* According to Fredrickson, *"To flourish emotionally, you need a 3-to-1 ratio. Three positive emotions for every negative one. Only 20 percent of Americans fall into that category, which means 80 percent do not. Even worse, almost 25 percent of Americans experience no life enjoyment at all!"*

Supporting the immune system through a healthy diet, proper sleep, stress reduction, appropriate exercise, not smoking or drinking alcohol, can keep the herpes predator wishing and hoping that we relapse.

Sleep

Sleep rejuvenates the immune system. While sleep requirements vary from person to person, most healthy adults need about 7 to 9 hours of sleep a night to function at their best. Children and teens need more. Increasing sleep can result in herpes outbreaks decreasing and/or often disappearing. Improve the quality of your sleep:

1. Leave work at the office, the office at work.
2. After 8 PM turn cell phones OFF or airplane mode.
3. Avoid popping sleeping pills like Ambien, instead try melatonin.
4. Give the eyes & mind a chance to unwind.
5. "Wind down" an hour before going to bed.
6. Cut off electronic and media devices.

Herpes and Exercise

Exercise floods the body with feel-good endorphins that activate opiate receptors. They in turn reduce physical tension, alleviate stress, benefit depression, lighten anxiety, and facilitate better sleep. Yoga, Qigong, and Tai Chi are uniquely effective at reducing stress because they combine exercise and meditation.

Regular exercise enhances the immune system, helping to prevent and fight infections. It also supports heart disease, cancer, and osteoporosis.

However, the intensity of exercise needs to be moderate to achieve this effect. Regular moderate-intensity exercise enhances, while strenuous, repetitive high-intensity exercise suppresses the immune system. To learn more how exercise can affect your immunity, copy the following hyperlink in your browser. https://bit.ly/3NXIoAW

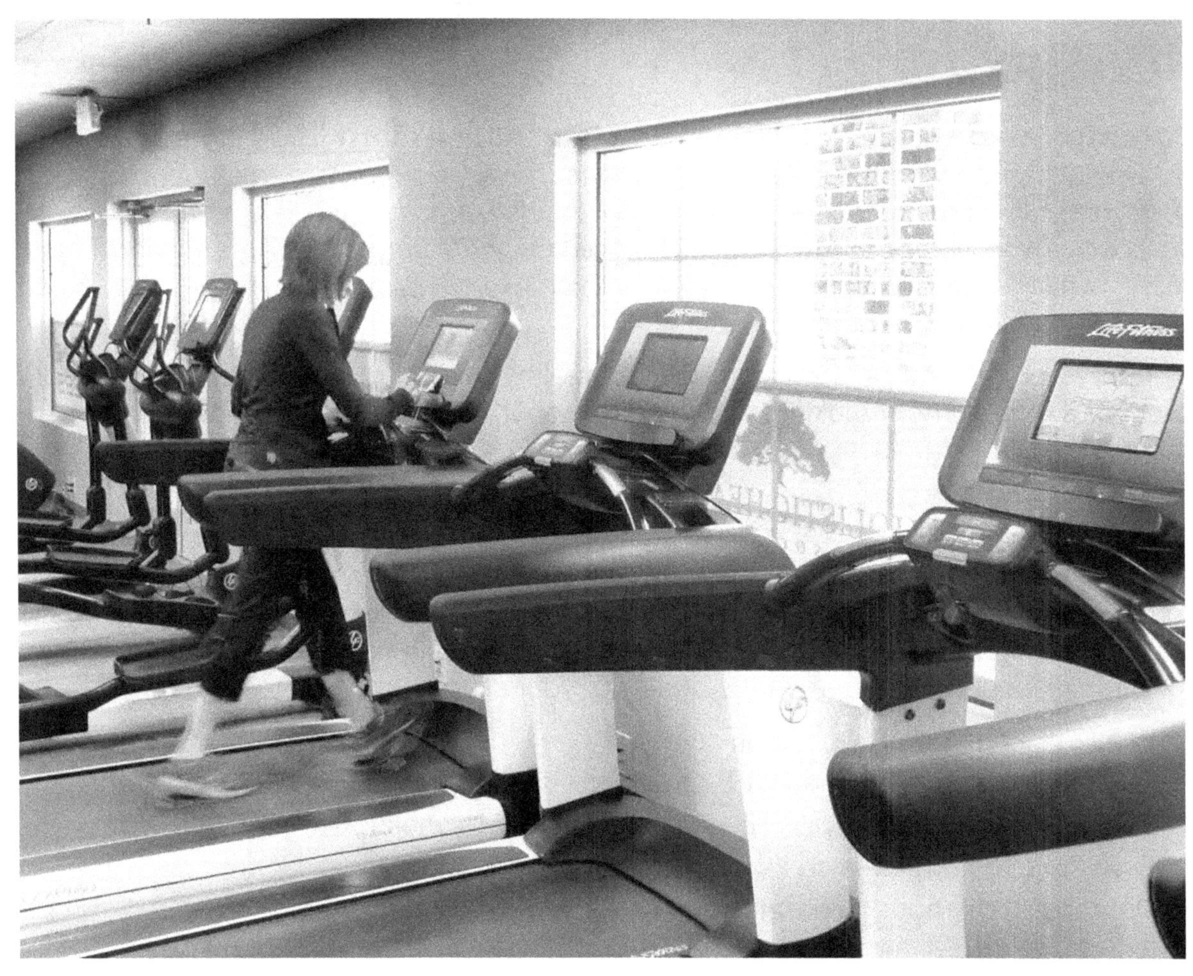

Chapter 8: Protocols

The Hermes Protocol is based on:

1. Clinical observations
2. Diet and nutrition
3. Psychological remedies
4. Alternative protocols
5. Immune support supplements
6. Decreasing the body's toxicity load.
7. Hair Tissue Mineral Analysis **(HTMA)** https://bit.ly/3Rogil9

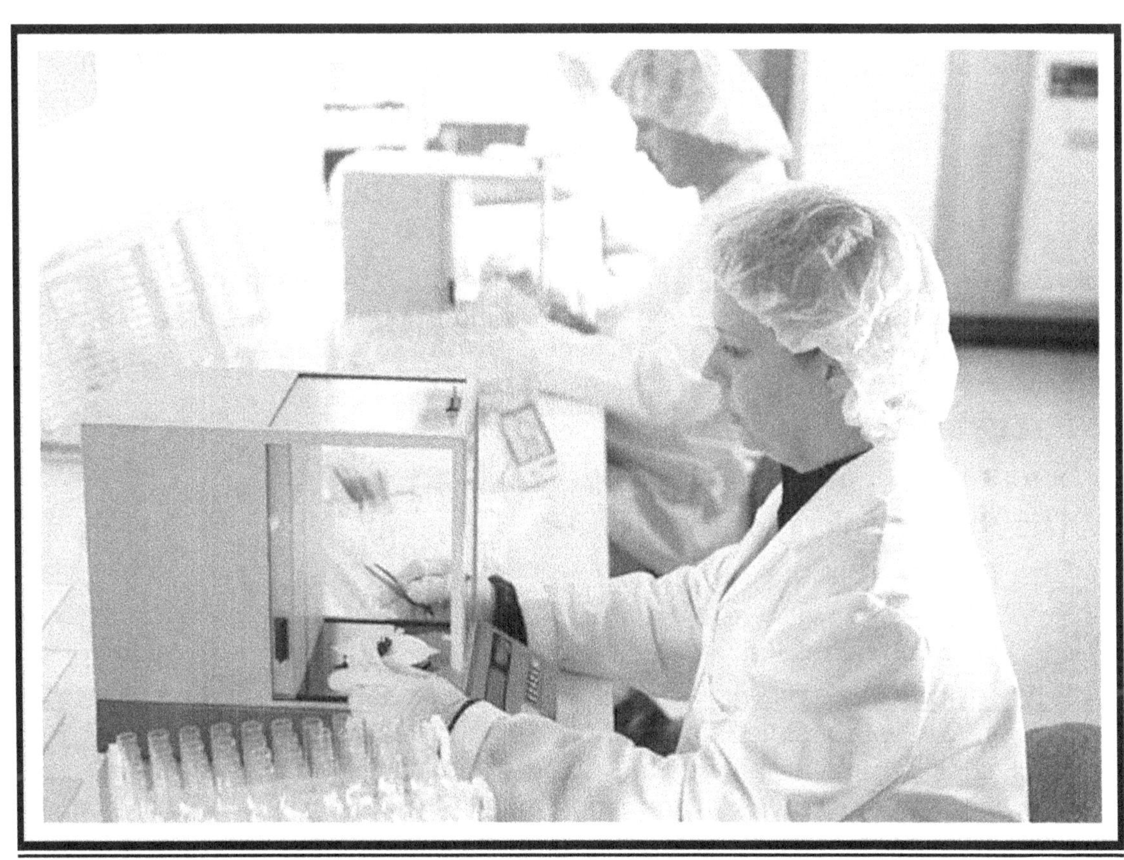

Physical remedies support the immune system to suppress outbreaks.

Psychological remedies attend emotional and mental well-being. They make physical remedies more effective.

Combined, they are greater than the sum of their parts in gaining the upper hand against Genital Herpes. Do not underestimate the power of your mind.

Familiarize yourself with each Physical and Psychological Remedy to see which ones resonate with you. Be cautious before adding supplements without a Hair Tissue Mineral Analysis (HTMA). It may compromise an already imbalanced profile. Then consider your financial resources and determine what's affordable. HTMA results pinpoint obvious toxicity and deficiency issues. Follow recommendations based on your toxic load and nutritional-vitamin-mineral status. **HTMA** kits can be ordered through:

Robert Thompson, M.D. Trace Elements, Inc.
www.aurorahealthandnutrition.com

Lawrence Wilson, M.D. at www.DrLWilson.com
Analytical Research Labs, Inc.

Vitamin and mineral supplements are one part of the Hermes Protocol. That and a proper diet are a good starting line. Remember, not every protocol will work the same for everyone. Like fingerprints, we are unique in our constitution. Please review all protocols and remedies in the next sections before making any decisions.

A. The Beck Protocol

Dr. Bob Beck's Protocol is an effective alternative practice. It supports the immune system and cleanses the body of infectious agents, including the herpes virus. There are four steps to the Becks Protocol that he developed from 1991 to 1997:

1. **First step** is *Micro-Pulsing*.
2. **The second,** *Magnetic Pulsing.*
3. **The third,** drinking *colloidal silver.*
4. **The fourth,** drinking *ozonated water.*

The Beck Protocol reconciles a wide variety of health challenges. Watch as Dr. Beck http://bit.ly/2np6HOT explains the *"Beck Protocol"* on YouTube. Enjoy this brilliant, compassionate genius translate into plain words how electricity heals the body. Because the herpes virus does not travel through the bloodstream, but along nerve fibers, it's difficult to treat. Any trauma to the nerves of the skin, such as a sunburn, fever, or even the flu can trigger a herpes or eczema outbreak.

The Beck Protocol is recommended as a stand-alone protocol for herpes. If outbreaks continue after several weeks of treatment, there may be other factors compromising the immune system: lifestyle choices, systemic candida infection, or hormonal issues. If there are a lot of toxins and pathogens in the body, the Beck Protocol will get their attention and they'll start looking for a more hospitable environment. To them you're now the HP Titanic, and the Beck Protocol has given them an ultimatum: *"Jump ship or die."*

Common Side Effects

Our skin is the body's largest elimination organ, where rashes, pimples, and even boils with puss can develop. The locations vary, but the more distressing ones are on the face. This is not a bad sign; it just means that the Beck Protocol is working to kill herpes. If a person feels too sick, back off. Give the liver and kidneys a couple of days rest. Then start again with a smaller, slower, and longer build-up time. Don't overburden the liver and kidneys. Detoxification is not a 100-meter hurdle, but a marathon.

There is conflicting information whether colloidal silver and ozonated water kill the "good" microbes in our intestinal tract. I error on the side of caution and add probiotics to nourish and replenish the "friendly" gut bacteria whenever I use any part of the Beck Protocol.

Daily Schedule after 5 PM

Weekends are more flexible. Remember, add a teaspoon of sea salt to any purified or spring water for the necessary electrolytes required by the Magnetic Pulser. Try to squeeze dinner in before drinking the allocated water, and/or before Blood Purification.

5:00 PM	Drink ozonated water, with electrolytes (e.g., sea salt).
5:30 PM	Drink more ozonated water.
6:00 PM	Start Magnetic Pulsing.
7:00 PM	Finish Magnetic Pulser.
7:00 PM	Start Blood Purification.
9:00 PM	Finish Blood Purifier.
9:30 PM	Drink Colloidal Silver, take supplements.

Finish both electro-medicine treatments before taking any supplements or colloidal silver. While the Beck Protocol takes significant time, it's possible to continue most normal activities during its schedule. For complete instructions please read My Friend, the Enemy: Genital Herpes.

PEMF (Pulsating Electro Magnetic Field) Therapy

The science behind PEMF has to do with your mitochondria—the battery packs of the body's cells. They affect the health of the entire body. With PEMF therapy you are basically "charging" your mitochondria directly or plugging them in and using bursts of low-level-electromagnetic radiation to heal damaged tissue and stimulate organs.

The healing frequencies of PEMF (Magnetic Pulsing) are like the frequencies you find in nature, so your body is familiar and knows how to allocate them. According to Dr. Gary Ryan, and Dr. Pawluck, both PEMF experts, *"based on research at Yale, it is apparent that just about any pathology in the body is preceded by a drop in cell charge. Now we have a technology that will reach down to the level of a cell that has lost charge and, due to the high intensity of the pulse, bring that pulse back to normal or a more natural situation, which allows it to replicate and produce a more normal cell."*

The body then uses that energy to heal itself through its natural healing mechanism, instead of using toxic drugs. The author bought a PEMF unit from Dr. Pawluck and used it effectively to heal damaged and broken skin from eczema, herpes, and Herpeticum.

The MAS Special Multi + is based on research from the Technical University of Munich in Germany. Since the earth has a pulse frequency around ten pulses per second, test subjects in Germany showed that if the earth's natural magnetic resonant field was removed, their health quickly deteriorated. To reverse that process, a frequency generator was used to introduce artificial magnetic fields into the test chamber, and it was discovered that 7.83 hertz was the ideal frequency to support life. The 7.83 frequency, thereafter, became known as the Schumann Resonance after its discoverer. Please visit https://www.drpawluk.com/ to learn more.

I place the MAS PEMF mat on a massage table for full body treatment and the pillow for targeted treatment. The **MAS Special Multi+** has 94 fully programmable settings that gives you the opportunity to regenerate your body. The program group *"Wellness"* can support the health of your being, and I use these programs almost every day to feel better and more energized.

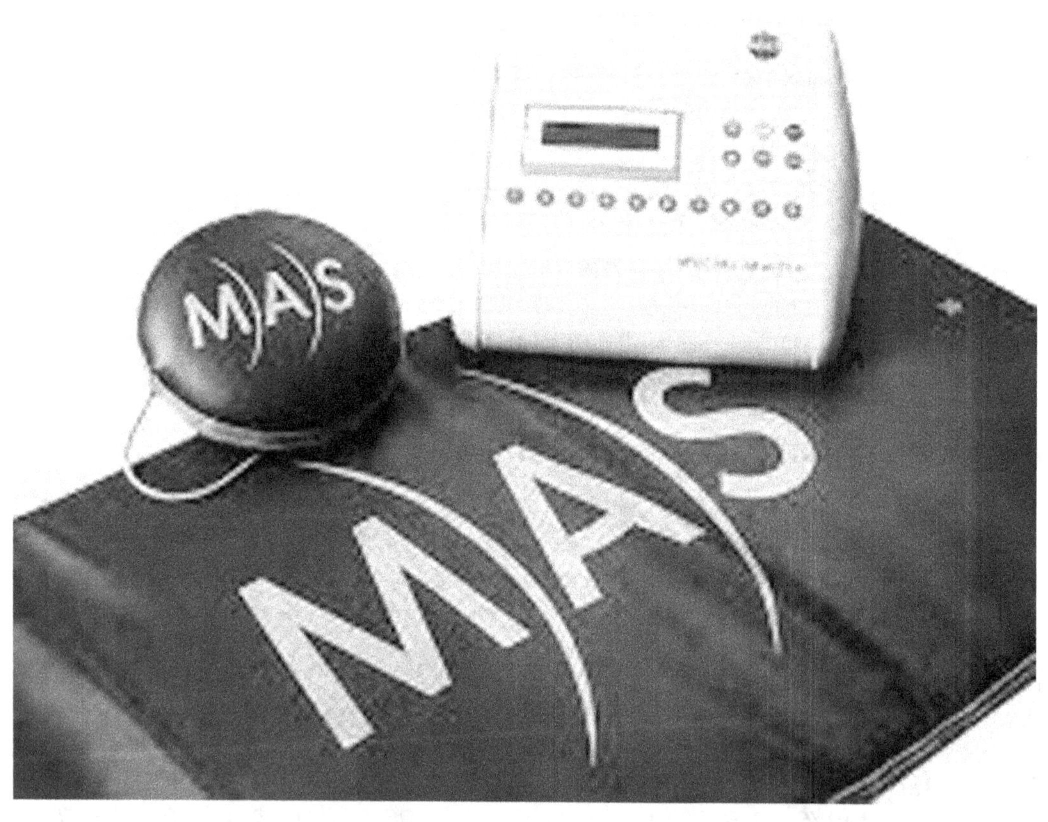

B. Colloidal Silver

Colloidal Silver is a favorite supplement for many, and I want to elaborate on its benefits, misperceptions, and as a stand-alone protocol. The internet "gurus" talk about how easy it is to make "clean-and-pure" colloidal silver. It's only partially true, and also borrowed-big-box marketing hype. Making colloidal silver is not as easy as their "plug-and-play" propaganda want you to believe. It's not difficult, but it does take time and requires your attentiveness. There are also as many manufacturers as there are claims that theirs is the only "pure" and "best" colloidal silver on the market. More marketing duplicity.

According to www.SilverSafety.org *"All products called ionic silver, colloidal silver, nano silver, hydrosol, or mild silver protein, are in fact just various forms of ionic silver. They all function by providing a delivery mechanism to release silver ions in the body. Otherwise, they would be useless."* So, if you hear, read, or are told that one type of colloidal silver is better than the other, go to the Silver Safety Council's website to read their non-biased opinion.

Also, when it comes to PPM or 'parts per million,' there is no such things as a "safer" level of PPM, just as there is no such thing as a more "effective" level of PPM. PPM is literally nothing more than a measure of how much water you're getting with the silver.

"Colloidal silver is a completely natural, liquid mineral supplement found in almost every health food store in North America. It is much like mineral water, except that in this case, the only minerals in the water are tiny, sub-microscopic particles of pure silver. Pure silver, by itself, has been known for thousands of years to have powerful, broad-spectrum infection-fighting qualities. So, when the process for making colloidal silver was discovered in the late 1800s, shortly after Edison harnessed electricity, it immediately became a popular natural infection-fighting agent, used both topically on cuts, burns and infections, and internally as a remedy for a wide variety of infectious diseases." Life & Health Research Group, LLC, PO Box 1239, Peoria AZ 85380-1239. https://lifeandhealthresearchgroup.com

Benefits of Colloidal Silver

1. **Anti-Bacterial:** colloidal silver's unique ability to control antibiotic-resistant superbugs is astonishing. UCLA Medical School documented over 650 different disease-causing pathogens that were destroyed in minutes when exposed to small amounts of silver. Unlike antibiotics, it doesn't create resistance (to-date) in the "bugs" that it kills. That's a good thing, since we are at the end-stage of a serious antibiotic-resistant epidemic. In 2013 the (CDC) reported each year more than 2 million people in the U.S. suffer because of antibiotic-resistant infections, and 23,000 of those die. https://bit.ly/3c7Pl5j

2. **Antiviral:** few will argue that colloidal silver is a powerful natural antibacterial and antifungal agent. But its ability to protect against viruses has not been embraced by the medical community until recently.

3. **In June 2005,** the journal, *Nanobiotechnology* published a 10-page study called: ***Interaction of silver nanoparticles with HIV-1*** which demonstrated in test tubes that silver nanoparticles inhibited the AIDS virus from binding to host cells. http://bit.ly/2noM1pb

When researchers placed the AIDS virus alongside human cells, silver particles stopped viral infection from taking place. In addition to HIV/AIDS, colloidal silver is an effective antiviral for pneumonia, herpes, shingles, warts, and against hepatitis C. All microbes, including viruses, need specific enzymes to help them live. Colloidal silver disables them, and therefore, Genital Herpes cannot survive. Colloidal silver is not a cure-all for herpes, but an effective treatment orally, topically, and as a rinse.

The Blues

Do you ever get the blues? Probably not like Paul Karason, or "Papa Smurf," as he was affectionately called. Papa Smurf had a condition called *Argyria.* It's where a person's skin turns a greyish blue by over ingesting certain silver preparations. Colloidal silver did **NOT** cause this disorder, as many pharmaceutical Trojans, the media, or FDA watchdog proponents want you to believe.

Infamously known as the *"blue-man,"* Paul Karason drank 700 ml, or almost 3/4 of a quart of silver a day before his skin turned blue. Yet it took 14 years. A rare individual among more than ten million users who've ever complained of any negative side effect. But it wasn't *colloidal* silver that turned him blue. **The "blue-man" effect** was not caused by ingesting *colloidal* silver as is often misrepresented. Karason made his own silver mixture using **salts** to generate a **silver chloride solution** with large silver particles. This high-risk blend is far different from the colloidal silver solutions sold at stores or that you can make at home.

In 2009 a coalition of environmentalists funded by major drug companies declared that nano-silver should be declared a "pesticide." It turned out "not to be," but that doesn't mean it won't resurface. http://bit.ly/2nqtSr8

There is a way to make your own high-quality colloidal silver. Two options to consider: the **Micro Particle** Colloidal Silver Generator (see below) from www.TheSilverEdge.com, or the **Silver Gen** Colloidal Silver Generator from www.silvergen.com.

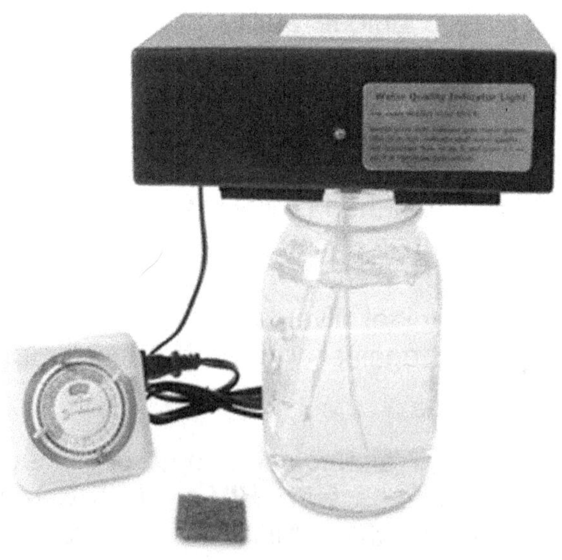

Homeopathy

Homeopathy embraces a natural approach to the treatment of disease. Founded in Germany in the late 1700s, it's still practiced throughout Europe. Homeopathy literally means *"like-disease,"* and the prescribed medicine is *"like-the-disease"* expressed.

Compared to Western medicine's annihilation mantra of *"drugs-radiation-and-surgery,"* or, to "eliminate" disease with a foreign or "unrelated" treatment. In homeopathy remedies are diluted and concentrated into a tincture of natural substances. Again-and-again the tincture or remedy is diluted. With repeated dilution, the physical characteristics are diminished, but their energetic healing properties are actually increased. The higher the dilution, the more potent a remedy, and the greater its healing power.

Homeopathy also has a compelling safety history that includes children, pregnant and nursing women, and senior citizens. Side effects are rare but occur if too much of the correct remedy is used too frequently. Known as "homeopathic aggravation," it's generally self-limiting, or can be relieved by drinking a strong cup of coffee. Which is something you don't want to do within a half-hour before or after taking a homeopathy remedy. It's also recommended that you do not to eat or drink anything within that 30-minute window.

A rule of thumb, the more acute and severe the symptoms, the more often the remedy is prescribed. In the initial stages, the "pellets" are sometimes used every 15 minutes, then tapered off as symptoms subside.

Homeopathy for Genital Herpes

Homeopathic remedies are tiny *"pellets"* of energy released when dissolved under the tongue. It's quite simple: pour the desired number of pellets into the cap and pop them under the tongue. Try not touch or handle the pellets directly. Some instructions recommend taking five to ten pellets, but often it's not necessary to take more than four or five. The number of pellets is not as important as the frequency of the dose. For example, with chronic Genital Herpes the length of treatment is more significant, whereas, in acute cases with severe symptoms the frequency is important.

C. Cell Salts

Wilhelm H. Schuessler, another German doctor, in the late 1800s discovered twelve (12) inorganic mineral salts after analyzing the *"ash-residue"* of human cells. He determined that numerous diseases are a deficiency or imbalance in these Cell-Salts, and with proper supplementation the body would heal itself.

Cell-Salts are unique because they're absorbed by the mucous membranes (mouth) and not the body's digestive system. The irony, many diseases have their origin in poor digestion. If that's the case, it doesn't matter whether you eat organic, Happy Meals, or supplement with the most natural, expensive vitamins.

If the body can't digest or absorb their nutrients, it will continue to be in a state of deficiency and ill health. Made from inorganic minerals, Cell-Salts can be taken without concern of toxicity, overdosing, or allergic reactions. In fact, Schuessler Salts are often used to treat allergies caused by mineral deficiencies or a defective metabolism. Cell Salts have a long history of safety and do not interfere with traditional medications, because they're absorbed at the cell-level and not through digestion. They can also be added to a bottle of water and sipped throughout the day. Best of all, they're baby and 'Fido' safe.

Cell-Salts are less complicated than traditional homeopathy. There are only twelve basic salts, compared to several thousand homeopathic formulations. Since Dr. Schuessler's discovery, an additional fifteen salts have been verified; however, most treatments use the original twelve salts. Schuessler salts are numbered from one to twelve, but American 'ego-nuity' uses a different numbering system than the rest of the world. Not a big deal unless you're reading, learning, traveling, or ordering products from the rest of the world. Always double check *their names, not numbers*.

For over 130 years, millions of people worldwide have used Cell-Salts. They have proved helpful in balancing many conditions, including Genital Herpes. Salts are an equilibrium remedy that balances the body's excess and/or deficiencies. They're often referred to as the "vitamins & minerals" of homeopathy. For supporting a chronic condition, like Genital Herpes, take a Cell-Salt remedy for 6 months or up to a year.

The 12 Cell-Salts

1. **Calcarea fluor** (Calcium fluoride) #1
2. **Calcium phos** (Calcium phosphate) #2
3. **Calcium sulph** (Plaster of Paris) #3
4. **Ferrum phos** (Iron phosphate) #4
5. **Kali mur** (Potassium chloride) #5
6. **Kali phos** (Potassium phosphate) #6
7. **Kali sulf** (Potassium sulphate) #7
8. **Magnesia phos** (Magnesium phosphate) #8
9. **Natrum mur** (Sodium chloride) #9
10. **Natrum sulf** (Sodium sulphate) #10
11. **Natrum phos** (Sodium phosphate) #11
12. **Silicea** (Silica) #12

Bioplasma

Not sure how to treat an under-performing immune system or Genital Herpes? Start with Bioplasma. It includes all 12 Cell-Salts and is manufactured either in tablets or a sport's drink used by athletes. Luyties Bioplasma comes in 500 tablet bottles and can be in 6x or 30x potency. Hylands Bioplasma comes in a 500 or 1000 tablet bottles and in a standard combination of 6x and 3x potencies. Both can be found on Amazon.com.

Herpes Cell-Salts Protocol

After several months of dosing with Bioplasma, I started the 1st Cell-Salts treatment:

1. **Kali mur, #5**
2. **Kali phos, #6**
3. **Nat mur, #9**

When things calmed down, I switched to the 2nd Cell-Salts phase:

1. **Silicea, #12**
2. **Calc Sulph, #3**

Dose and Frequency: during an active herpes outbreak, take five tablets, four times a day. Each tablet measures one grain. When two or more Cell-Salts are used, rotate them every two hours. In acute cases, a dose every 1/2 hour may be needed, but for no more than a day or two. Thereafter, the dose is back to three or four times per day. Long-term dosing for chronic herpes infections is two or three doses daily for several months.

Put the tablets underneath the tongue and wait for them to dissolve. Do not take strong spices, stimulants like coffee, tea, tobacco, or wine within 30 minutes of dosing Cell-Salt remedies. No Salts within one hour before or after meals. Taking Cell-Salts may initially aggravate detox symptoms. Headaches, slight fever, or skin issues are common. Don't get frustrated or upset. It may indicate the healing force inside your body has been stimulated. Back off if it's too intense.

Give Cell-Salts Time: to correct deficiencies so the immune system can do its job. Results are not as fast as traditional medicine but are safer, longer lasting, and improve immune function.

D. DMSO

April 3, 1963, the *New York Times* called DMSO the closest thing to a wonder drug, until the FDA took if off the shelves. Discovered in 1886, DMSO (Dimethyl Sulfoxide) is an organic sulfur, a by-product of manufacturing paper. In 1959 scientists discovered that DMSO protected red blood cells and transplant tissue from freezing. That started the practice of preserving donor organs with DMSO. Today, DMSO is still used for preservation of transplant organs. One of its many uses.

Many are familiar with the supplement MSM or Methylsulfonylmethane, an organic sulfur compound derived from DMSO. It's used for joint, allergy, and gut health. MSM has many of the same properties as DMSO but is not considered as effective. But then MSM has very little controversy surrounding its use, while DMSO has been called *"the most controversial therapeutic advance of modern times."* The controversy seems to be more bureaucratic and economic, rather than scientific.

DMSO was the first nonsteroidal anti-inflammatory discovered since aspirin. That breakthrough drove pharmaceutical companies to develop other nonsteroidal anti-inflammatories. They intuitively knew that if DMSO is so effective, then other *'manufactured'* and *'marketed'* compounds can also be, but *they'll patent them*. The irony, *"DMSO is less toxic and has fewer side effects."* The author has used DMSO successfully since 2011, internally and topically for herpes and Herpeticum, as well as a 40% eye drop solution.

In 1975, Dr. Robert Hill of Longview, Washington, reported his eyesight studies. *"Of the 50 DMSO treated patients, 22 had improved visual acuity, nine had improved visual fields and five improved in dark adaption. Only two patients out of the 50 continued to get worse. The remaining patients had no noticeable changes in vision. Without the treatment, it is probable that all 50 patients would have continued to regress."* http://bit.ly/2Eembel

The purity of DMSO is essential. Don't buy cheap knock-off brands. DMSO is also a vasodilator, which means it can increase blood flow. That's why so many athletes use it because it allows blood to reach football or basketball injuries that are difficult to treat. I'm confident that this book, like DMSO, will cross your brain barrier. Carry with it the information you need to treat Genital Herpes and progress *"To-Be-Herpes-Free."*

DMSO is an effective treatment for viral infections, including herpes. In 1971, Dr. William Campbell Douglas, MD, conducted a DMSO clinical study with 46 patients infected with shingles. He applied DMSO on their lesions at various strengths, from 50 percent to 90 percent. Some were only treated with DMSO; others combined DMSO with corticosteroid. There was no difference in the results, but this is important to remember for future applications: *"The best results were obtained with patients treated early in the disease."* http://bit.ly/2DLHS5G

IMPORTANT: The skin must be dry and clean from any contaminants. Use only 99.99% pharmaceutical grade DMSO. Dilute with distilled water to lower its concentrations. DMSO is an effective stand-alone **topical** treatment for herpes and/or Eczema Herpeticum, or as an **internal** option to support the immune system. Topical DMSO applications for herpes outbreaks and eczema flare-ups, depending on their location, can be from 50% to 90% liquid or gel strength. The liquid penetrates better; the gel is more easily mixed with other topicals. You can also combine colloidal silver or lemon balm cream with DMSO. Apply and leave on for about 20 minutes, then wipe off the rest. For more sensitive areas, reduce the DMSO % concentration.

E. High-Dose Vitamin-C

Herpes, Shingles, and Vitamin-C

Even as far back as 1936 scientists knew that vitamin-C was a possible treatment *for herpes infections.* http://bit.ly/2FvUyhv Research showed it to be a powerful virus-killing agent. The most impressive results of *high-dose-C* for shingles was published in 1950. Researchers reported a complete resolution in 327 out of 327 shingles patients treated with intravenous vitamin C, all within 72 hours from the start of treatment. http://bit.ly/2DWR6iS No side effects were recorded, other than the occasional loose stools and stinky "essential-oil-diffuser" moments.

It's hard to ignore the facts or "studies" of vitamin-C. If you search Pub Med, there are over 50,000 studies indexed in the medical literature on the extraordinary qualities of vitamin-C. So, if you ever hear there are no studies about the value of vitamin-C, it's a lie. There are just no *"positive"* studies funded by pharmaceutical interests. Like most other natural treatments, vitamin-C is held to a different and more complex standard than conventional treatments and prescription drugs.

The key for effective Vitamin-C therapy (orally or intravenously):

1. QUANTITY
2. FREQUENCY
3. DURATION

I've often heard, *"I shouldn't have to take so much vitamin-C."* That's maybe true, but for a quick recovery it's important to use it effectively. When it comes to Genital Herpes or any disease, I'm not interested in opinions, but results. So, remember, take what the body requires and wants, NOT what you *think* you need, or what you think you *should* take.

Which Form of Vitamin-C is Best?

1. **Liposomal absorption** is unlike intestinal absorption. It enters the cells directly. The fat layer of the liposome protects vitamin-C from coming in direct contact with the stomach and intestines. This protection prevents intestinal side effects and increases absorption from 20% to almost 80%.

2. **Mineral ascorbates** are the lion's share of vitamin-C. The most common are sodium ascorbate, calcium ascorbate, and magnesium ascorbate.

3. **Sodium ascorbate** may be the safest, and least expensive, for high-dose supplementation. Anecdotally, multi-gram doses of sodium ascorbate do not seem to adversely affect blood pressure. However, in biology there are exceptions to every rule. If you notice elevated blood pressures or ankle edema after high doses of sodium ascorbate, it would be well advised to supplement with a different form of vitamin-C.

4. **Calcium ascorbate is** a popular form of vitamin-C supplementation, but is best avoided. Excess calcium is directly correlated to an increased risk of heart attacks, chronic degenerative disease, and overall "all-cause mortality."

5. **Magnesium ascorbate** is bioavailable and effective throughout the body in reversing the damage done by excess calcium. As such, it is a valuable treatment for osteoporosis. While there is nothing wrong with taking magnesium ascorbate (unless you are hypothyroid), it's more economical to take sodium ascorbate.

6. **Potassium, manganese, zinc, molybdenum, and chromium** ascorbates are additional mineral ascorbates. However, they can be easily overdosed. I would avoid them.

7. **Ascorbyl palmitate** is a fat-soluble form of vitamin-C and is absorbed into the cell membrane where ascorbic acid cannot reach. It is also retained in the body for a longer period. Ascorbyl palmitate is an amphipathic molecule, which means one end is water-soluble, the other fat-soluble. *"This dual solubility allows it to permeate the extra-cellular aqueous environment of the cell and the interior cellular environment, as well. When it is incorporated into the cell membranes of human red blood cells, ascorbyl palmitate protects them from oxidative damage and helps protect vitamin E (a fat-soluble antioxidant) from oxidation by free radicals."* Ascorbyl palmitate is an expensive way to provide multi-gram doses of ascorbate.

Current Recommendations

How do you determine what the body needs? I'm glad you asked. According to Dr. Levy, MD, *"Although far from perfect, one of these mechanisms, bowel tolerance, is a good starting point."* In other words, if you experience loose stools, without diarrhea, you've reached tolerance.

Please remember, liposome vitamin-C enjoys nearly complete absorption. It will not cause a diarrheal flush. It is considerably more bioavailable. The following substitution schedule provides approximate values:

1,000 mg liposomal = 3,000 -- 4,000 mg powder

2,000 mg liposomal = 8,000 -- 10,000 mg powder

3,000 mg liposomal = 12,000 -- 18,000 mg powder

As I mentioned earlier, I do not recommend calcium ascorbate. While many people want to avoid the *"C-flush"* effect, or intestinal discomfort, every so often it's a good way to keep the gut detoxified and clean. For those wishing to have near-complete vitamin "C" absorption, the liposome-encapsulated and "very expensive form" of vitamin-C is optimal.

Safety, Side Effects & Myths

The safety of vitamin-C is **extraordinary.** There is not one case of vitamin-C toxicity anywhere in the world's medical literature. Frederick R. Klenner, MD, of North Carolina cured diphtheria, staph and strep infections, ***herpes***, mumps, spinal meningitis, mononucleosis, shock, viral hepatitis, arthritis, and polio using high doses of vitamin-C. According to Dr. Klenner, *"Ascorbic acid is the safest and the most valuable substance available to the physician,"* and *"If you want results, use adequate ascorbic acid."* http://bit.ly/2EryXaV

What do guinea pigs, fruit bats, gorilla's, lemurs, and New York City dwellers have in common? Besides downright obnoxious at times, they **cannot** produce their own vitamin-C.

1. Humans
2. Primates
3. Guinea Pigs
4. Fruit Bats

While the USDA daily recommended allowance for vitamin-C is **90 mg**, all other mammals on average consume between 3,000 to 11,000 mg. per day. The fact that the guinea pig cannot make vitamin-C is one of the reasons it has served science so well. *"MMmmm, I wonder? Guinea pigs? Humans? Who's the real guinea when it comes to scientific quackery called research? Naw, they wouldn't."*

So, at 90 mg you live. At moderate consumption of 500 to 1,500 mg you build health, have fewer colds, and flu severity will be less. But at 8,000 to 40,000 mg per day it has therapeutic properties: antihistamine, antitoxin, antibiotic, and antiviral. It may be an excellent adjunct to other Herpeticum protocols. The author has consumed on average 10,000 mg per day for many years and has not had the flu or cold during that time.

Vitamin-C works like money and gasoline. Money buys things. Even if you have a lot of it, its nature does not change. But its power does. And if it takes 111 gallons of gas to drive 2,789 miles from New York City to Los Angeles, you're not going to make it on 70 gallons. No matter how hard you try. Likewise, if the body wants 40,000 mg of vitamin-C to fight an infection, 6,000 mg won't do. The key to vitamin-C supplementation is taking enough, often enough, and long enough.

A word of caution for those with kidney disease or compromised renal function. It is essential you work with a qualified health practitioner before dosing with vitamin-C. Also, if you've been taking calcium supplements for years, without extra vitamin K-2, it's possible that extensive calcium deposits have accumulated throughout the body, including your arteries. Vitamin-C dissolves calcium, so when a person starts taking C for the first time, greater amounts of calcium will be dissolved. Stay well hydrated and start with smaller doses of vitamin-C. Increase your dose slowly over time. For those seeking objective measurements, get a *periodic urinary calcium measurement test* from your doctor. It indicates the amount of calcium being excreted from the body. Once that's stabilized, then increase the vitamin-C dose. Also, if you have ANY medical condition that needs to be treated and monitored, always check with your health care provider before taking higher doses of C or any vitamin.

Ascorbic Acid is the straight form of vitamin-C and is not buffered. It can aggravate the stomach, especially for those with GI issues, such as GERD or ulcers. A buffered form of vitamin-C, like Sodium Ascorbate is ideal for mega-dosing.

WARNING: large doses of vitamin-C are contraindicated with certain blood diseases including *sickle-cell anemia, hemochromatosis, and thalassemia.* The following are also consideration to keep in mind:

1. **Vitamin-C** increases iron and decreases copper absorption.

2. **Ascorbic Acid,** the acid form of vitamin-C, may aggravate stomach ulcers.

3. **Ascorbic Acid** can cause diarrhea, which may NOT be a desired outcome.

4. **A myth** that is often bantered about as truth is that large doses of vitamin-C trigger kidney stones. To date it has never been proven, documented, or substantiated, but is often quoted by critics of vitamin-C. The evidence indicates this claim is false.

5. **Other myths,** but my favorite is that vitamin-C increases the risk of cancer. The irony, the latest cancer research shows just the opposite http://bit.ly/2GxjOVV.

F. Low Dose Naltrexone (LDN)

Forty years ago, two researchers from Penn State University, Drs. Ian Zagon and Pat McLaughlin, discovered that Low Dose Naltrexone (**LDN**) helped relieve symptoms of multiple sclerosis (MS). Since then, they've studied the effects of **LDN** on a wide range of diseases. For example, **Naltrexone** has been FDA approved to treat heroin addiction for over 20 years.

They use it in a 50-mg dose to *"block"* opioid receptors, so addicts can no longer get *"high."* From this idea, Drs. Zagon & McLaughlin, created Low Dose Naltrexone in a 3-to-4.5 mg dose. Research found it to be beneficial for autoimmune conditions such as lupus, rheumatoid arthritis, multiple sclerosis, and cancer, as well as infectious diseases such as HIV and Genital Herpes. http://bit.ly/2DMpOs0

LDN taken at bedtime boosts the immune system by stimulating the body's own natural defenses. Research studies indicate that endorphin secretions play a key role in modulating the immune system. LDN at bedtime blocks certain opioid receptors during the early morning hours (from 2 a.m. to 4 a.m.). Afterwards, it induces a prolonged up-regulation of the immune system. In plain immune armed forces dialogue, *"More good guys to fight the bad guys."*

Considering the impact of LDN on the immune system http://bit.ly/2EoosVO (YouTube), Genital Herpes may be influenced by LDN therapy. Talk to your "alternative" doctor or go to www.LDNscience.org to find one and learn more about the therapeutic benefits of LDN. It's *"the most credible up-to-date information website about Low Dose Naltrexone (LDN) for Physicians, Researchers, and Patients."*

G. Chlorine Dioxide

MMS + 4% Hydrochloric Acid = **Chlorine Dioxide (CD)**

Sodium Chlorite (MMS) + 4% HCl (Hydrochloric Acid) = MMS1 or (CD)

The above formulas are the same (but with different terminology) on how to make Chlorine Dioxide (CD). Or what Jim Humble refers to as MMS1. However, **Master Mineral Solution** or **MMS** are the terms most people use when talking about **Chlorine Dioxide,** even though technically it's not correct. Strictly speaking, the acronym MMS is un-activated 22.4% Sodium Chlorite solution (NaClO2) in water. Not Chlorine Dioxide, which is MMS1.

Chlorine Dioxide and MMS1 are interchangeable terms for activated MMS. See table below for a more visual explanation. Take your time reading this condensed explanation of MMS. It's a simple subject muddied by acronyms, chemistry, and terminology, making it more confusing than it is. Absorb as much as you can, and then take advantage of the many internet blogs to learn more. If you can't recall formulas, MMS names, solutions, or acronyms, refer to this page for an abbreviated description.

1. **Sodium Chlorite** = Inactivated MMS or Master Mineral Solution (MMS)
2. **Un-activated MMS** = 22.4% solution of Sodium Chlorite (NaCl02)
3. **Activated MMS** = MMS1 or Chlorine Dioxide
4. **Chlorine Dioxide** = MMS1 and is often referred to as "activated" MMS

Most readers may not be familiar with the terms Sodium Chlorite or Chlorine Dioxide (CD) but may have heard the acronyms MMS or Master Mineral Solution. It's the label Jim Humble attached to un-activated MMS. He thought it was "miraculous" that MMS saved the life of a friend dying from malaria.

Chlorine Dioxide and MMS1 are the same solution. One is the technical name, the other a popularized version coined by Jim Humble. The internet is bursting with MMS testimonials from every part of the globe. Many in writing, more in video format. But there are also many *"quack-monials"* from those who have a vested-interest in seeing MMS fear-mongered. Hoping people will become too confused and afraid. Their favorite smear-tactic is: *"Would you drink bleach?"* Of course not, who would be that Wikipedia? But then Chlorine Dioxide is not chlorine. Like sodium chloride is not Sodium Chlorite. One is table salt. Which one? The one with the letter **"d."** Trying to discredit MMS by saying it's "bleach," is like saying water buffalos come from chickens. Yes, they are both alive, made up of living cells, and use energy. But they come from different genetic planets. Earth to Mars. Come in.

MMS1/Chlorine Dioxide (ClO2) and table salt (NaCl) both have the chlorine element in their composition. The "Cl" stands for chlorine. But the chlorine is not dangerous. Unless you consider table salt poison. Yet the FDA and the medical establishment keep slandering and attacking MMS with simple minded, uninformed scare tactics that doesn't hold up to 6th grade chemistry. By now I should be blind and look like Edward Scissorhands from doing laundry. The only thing I've ever felt is smarmy. Not even skin burns.

They use the word *"industrial"* bleach because it makes it sound dangerous. Think about it, most things are made in factories, an industry. There's nothing inherently bad about being industrial. It's manufactured marketing.

MMS Chemistry or Making MMS1:

1. **Start with Sodium Chlorite** (un-activated MMS). Do not ingest.
2. **Activate Sodium Chlorite** (MMS) with 4% HCl, hydrochloric acid.
3. **Wait about 90 seconds.** It turns into Chlorine Dioxide, or MMS1.
4. **Chlorine Dioxide (CD)** is the technical term for MMS1.

You may have used Chlorine Dioxide and not even known it. The following products contain Chlorine Dioxide approved by the Food and Drug Administration (FDA). They are manufactured by Frontier Pharmaceutical, Alcide, Bioxy, and others for skin and oral care:

1. Cankers Away
2. DioxiRinse™ Mouthwash
3. DioxiBrite™ Toothpaste
4. DioxiWhite™ Pro Teeth Whitener

5. WhiteLasting™ Maintenance Gel
6. BioClenz™ Dental Unit Waterline Cleaner
7. Penetrator™ Periodontal Gel
8. Simply Clear™ Acne Treatment

History

Millions have used and benefited from MMS1 worldwide. There is an MMS documentary www.quantumleap.is and a YouTube video of the history of the Genesis II Church. http://bit.ly/2Gsx91E

Chlorine Dioxide is a free radical, so antioxidants quench it back into a chlorite form. Do not consume antioxidant supplements, natural juices, or rich antioxidant foods while taking MMS. Lemon or lime juice has vitamin-C, so they're not a good mix either. Other antioxidants to avoid include vitamins E, A, CoQ10, flavonoids, Beta-carotene, Lycopene, and Lutein.

DO NOT MAKE Sodium Chlorite on your own. Buy Sodium Chlorite and the 4% Hydrochloric Acid activator from a reputable company. Here's a list of approved "water purification" vendors http://www.wpsuppliers.com.

Dosage

Large internal doses of MMS1 may cause nausea, vomiting or diarrhea. This is probably not a Herxheimer reaction, but the body's attempt to get rid of MMS1. I've not experienced those symptoms, but other people have. There is a significant benefit from taking low dose MMS1. It stimulates white blood cells to produce cytokines. They in turn stimulate other white blood cells, thereby activating the immune system. Another MMS1 benefit is that it destroys most venom and poisons. Compared to anti-venoms that cost $10,000, have a short shelf life, and hospitals seldom stock, it may be wise for that reason alone to keep some MMS and an activator handy.

Starting *Internal* Protocol

Jim Humble suggests that everyone start out at 1/4 drop of MMS1. The "new" three golden rules of dosing a 1/4 drop every hour:

1. **If you are getting better,** don't change anything.
2. **If you are feeling worse,** cut your next dose in half.
3. **If not feeling worse or better** (nothing has changed) increase the dose.

WARNING: keep MMS out of the reach of children and pets, and **DO NOT** keep it in unmarked bottles or glass. MMS has no smell and is almost impossible to tell apart from water. Some have drunk as much as 1/2 a glass of MMS before realizing they were not drinking water.

If you drink too much MMS, either by mistake or on purpose, immediately drink as much water with salt as possible. Try to induce vomiting. Use one tablespoon of salt per one liter or quart of water. Then drink more and try to vomit again. Do this several times. If you still feel bad, go to the hospital. Before using MMS as outlined in this book for Genital Herpes, read Jim Humble's book, *MMS Health Recovery Guidebook.* Click here www.mmsnews.is.

Topical MMS for Herpes, Eczema, or Herpeticum

1. Twenty (20) drops un-activated MMS in a 2-ounces glass spray bottle.

2. Add 20 drops of 4% HCL.

3. Wait 30 to 60 seconds (it's now activated--MMS1).

4. Wait 2 minutes and fill the 2-ounce spray bottle with distilled water.

5. You now have spray bottle solution that stays fresh for about 3 day.

6. Spray your rash, eczema, Herpeticum, every two or three hours all day long.

Some individuals may be sensitive to MMS and will experience stinging, burning, or pain. If it does pour out half the liquid (one ounce) and fill with distilled water. If it still stings, repeat the process again. Continue diluting until there is no stinging or pain. It's rare but can happen. Many testimonials speak of complete remission after 3 weeks of using protocol 1000 or 2000. Please see below.

Step One: Protocol 1000 (All MMS YouTube Videos no longer available. Account Terminated.) I wonder why?

1. **Always use an empty,** clean, dry, 4-ounce glass.

2. **Tilt the glass** or put a chip under one side. Drip the MMS drops into the lower side of the glass. Hold the dropper bottle or eye dropper straight up and down when releasing drops.

3. **Using a 4% solution of HCl,** add the same amount of activator drops on top of the MMS drops. For example, if you used 4 drops of MMS, add 4 drops of 4% HCl.

<u>**Step Two:**</u> YouTube <u>http://bit.ly/2no3te8</u> (Video Not Available)

Swirl the drops a little as you wait about 60 to 90 seconds. The mixture should turn amber and let off gas. Try not to inhale the MMS1 gas.

<u>**Step Three:**</u> Dr. Andreas Kalcker, (YouTube Not Available) <u>http://bit.ly/2FvO1U9</u>

1. **After the mixture turns amber**, add 4 ounces/120 ml of clean drinking water.

2. **Purified water is OK, distilled better**. If the taste of MMS1 is objectionable, some juices are fine if they don't contain harmful preservatives and/or added vitamin-C. These cancel out the effectiveness of MMS1.

3. **Never use tap water.** Some bottled waters contain fluoride, chlorine, and other harmful substance. Distilled water is a better choice.

4. **If you are taking 1 drop of MMS1**, pour off 3 ounces of water and drink 1 ounce.

5. **Drink the dose fresh**, in less than 1 minute.

Some people find the taste of MMS1 difficult to swallow. Pathogens in the body create an aversion to whatever threatens them as a survival mechanism. Keep a positive attitude and do the best you can. Read Jim Humble's book before using MMS1:

<u>https://jimhumble.co/bookstore</u>

Chapter 9: Supplements

Do you have a lobby? I don't, but then I live in a modest townhome. However, if you ever get a chance to visit a pharmaceutical company, they have enormous lobbies in CNN, the New York Times, college universities, scientific journals, and our watchdog, the FDA. It's called the *"Anti-Supplement Lobby."*

August 23, 2017, CNN Health posted the following piece of propaganda. *"High doses of vitamin B6 & B12 tied to lung cancer risk, study says."* The Advisory Board of the Orthomolecular Medicine News Service (OMNS) had this to say, **"It's a crock."** http://orthomolecular.org

Click on their website if *"you've had enough of vitamin-bashing newspaper, magazine and TV reports."* Sign up for the truth about vitamins. In their Jan 2017 edition, there's an article on the safety of supplements http://bit.ly/2GuC42k "No Deaths from Supplements." Please do not to be fooled by anti-supplement articles. Remember, the media is on alert for "fake scare stories." That way we'll impassively, yet fearfully, sit through all their manufactured commercials and buy the crap we don't need.

A. Immune Support Vitamins

Boosting your immune system with proper nutrition and supplements can reduce the frequency and duration of Genital Herpes outbreaks. Part of that insurance is to make sure the body has an adequate intake of:

1. Vitamin A
2. Zinc
3. Selenium
4. Vitamin E
5. Vitamin C
6. A multiple vitamin/mineral supplement

A low Arginine diet and proper stress management, absorbing adequate amounts of vitamins and minerals is vital. Then we can look at specific supplements that directly impact the immune system. Like all props to healing, the eventual goal is to have the immune system do the heavy lifting, keeping herpes dormant. Because of our individual differences, the difficulty is discovering an effective combination. That's the reason we do a Hair Tissue Mineral Analysis (HTMA). **These five (5) vitamins** are a good foundation.

1. **Vitamin A:** during an active outbreak take 25,000 to 50,000 IU daily for 7 days, then reduce the dosage to 15,000 IU for seven more. After that, take 10,000 IU daily. Use natural vitamin A only.

2. **Vitamin-C:** take 10,000 mg, or an amount equal to bowel tolerance, in divided doses. The upper limit will be different for each person. Then back off until stools are soft, but not runny. Consider taking this amount until the infection is almost healed; at that point back off and take 5,000 to 10,000 mg.

3. **Vitamin E:** take up to 400 IU per day of natural E with mixed tocopherols and tocotrienols.

4. **Zinc:** take 25 mg two times a day during an outbreak and recovery state. Thereafter, depending on copper status, take 15 to 25 mg per day for maintenance. A word of caution regarding zinc and copper. They are antagonists and decrease or block the absorption of the other. Supplement them at different times or days. The HTMA analysis is the best way to monitor zinc and copper levels.

5. **Selenium:** take 200 mcg per day.

B. Balancing Complements

Our immune system's primary role is to protect our body against infections. Supporting and enhancing the immune system is perhaps the most important step we can take to keep Genital Herpes dormant. This involves a health-promoting lifestyle, conscious stress management, exercise, diet, and may include the appropriate use of the following immune supporting complements.

Thymic Protein A

Nutrient deficiency is the most frequent cause of a depressed immune system. Part of that deficit is exasperated by eating large amounts of sugar, one of the most damaging and toxic foods for the immune system. Taking a good multi-vitamin/mineral, in addition to specific supplements, can offset nutrient deficiency. http://bit.ly/2npiCv2

To help stimulate T-Lymphocytes, immune compromised individuals often take **Thymic Protein A.** Restoring T-Lymphocytes, restores the immune system's ability to fight Genital Herpes infections. **Terry Beardsley, PhD,** an immunologist, and experimental biologist, discovered a biologically "intact" 500-amino chain protein that fits into T-4 cells receptor sites. It's the key that "turns on" and programs the cells to fight disease. Dr. Beardsley called his discovery Thymic-Protein-A (TPA). With its unique oral delivery system, degradation of the thymic protein is avoided in the stomach, a significant problem with some other over-the-counter oral thymic preparations. In 1997, he was awarded a US patent for both the Thymic-Protein-A molecule and its method of production.

Nutrition Review, Dr. Julian Whitaker stated http://bit.ly/2nqXQvb that Thymic-Protein-A *"is likely the most powerful natural stimulant of the immune system ever discovered."* When ill, as with active herpes lesions, he recommends taking three packets a day, taken sublingually. For a maintenance dose, one packet a day will help support an impaired immune system. Thymic-Protein-A is safe, with no adverse side effects noted in any dose.

Beta 1, 3 Glucan

The problem with orthodox antiviral medications, like Acyclovir or Valtrex, they target the herpes virus only when it starts replicating. Then a long-term regimen is often necessary to keep herpes under control. Antiviral meds kill the infected cells but killing a neuron to get rid of a herpes virus is like *"burning down a village to save it."*

A better approach would be to destroy the virus in its latent state, before it starts replicating and without damaging the infected cell. That's where Beta Glucan can help. Technically, Beta Glucan is what is called an *"immunomodulator."* It renders the immune system more successful in fighting the herpes virus. Beta Glucan does NOT *stimulate* the immune system the way Thymic Protein A stimulates T-Lymphocytes, but instead *modulates* or *activates* the immune system.

Dr. Vaclav Vetvicka, Ph.D. in his book on Beta Glucan said, *"There are other agents that stimulate the immune system. However, glucans are in a class apart, because those other agents can push the immune system to overstimulation. This means they can make matters worse in the case of auto-immune illnesses such as lupus, multiple sclerosis, rheumatoid arthritis, allergies, and yeast functions."* Beta Glucan is a safe all-natural fiber molecule and the most studied natural immunomodulator on the planet. It has many benefits, not only helping the immune system do a better job keeping herpes dormant, but also stopping other diseases from establishing a foothold in the body.

There have been thousands of Beta Glucan studies by universities, medical schools, teaching hospitals, and even Canada's defense department. They show it to be protective against infections, to lower cholesterol and blood sugar, reduce stress, increase antibody production, heal wounds, help radiation burns, treat diabetes, and prevent the spread of cancer.

In the past, this supplement was too expensive to be on anyone's radar. However, recent breakthroughs in manufacturing have made Beta Glucan supplement affordable to most anyone. **The only caution** if you are a transplant patient, or immunosuppressant, do not take Beta Glucan. Otherwise, to maximize its benefits, it should be taken on an empty stomach with water. Then wait at least 30 minutes before eating or drinking. During an active Genital Herpes outbreak, take between 1,000 and 3,000 mg per day. Then back off to 300 to 1,000 mg, depending on age and immune status. Side effects are rare but start slowly.

Colostrum and Lactoferrin

Lactoferrin is a key component of **bovine colostrum** and is six percent of the total protein in Colostrum-LD, a well-recognized and researched brand name. http://bit.ly/2DQTatC.

Colostrum is the *pre-milk fluid* produced by female mammals just before they give birth. Technically it's not milk, but it's often called the "first-milk" because it's obtained from the first milking after birth. Giving birth triggers colostrum production.

Colostrum-LD is safe, non-allergenic, and has no known side effects. It can be consumed in any quantity and is safe for adults, children, and pets. In India, where cows are still considered sacred, colostrum is delivered like regular milk. It's often the first medication people take when sick. The FDA considers lactoferrin a food and not a supplement. Their best "idiopathic" guess is that antiviral activities takes place somewhere in the gastro-intestinal tract, thereby supporting the immune system.

2004 lactoferricin HSV study showed, *"that bovine lactoferricin blocks herpes simplex virus binding by competing for receptor sites on target cells. However, this is apparently not the only mechanism that accounts for its anti-HSV activity."* http://bit.ly/2DYBUSi And a study in *Cellular and Molecular Life Sciences* 62(24):3002-3013 (2005), showed that lactoferrin and a peptide derived from lactoferrin, blocked entry of HSV into cells.

Dosage: for chronic herpes outbreaks it depends on the state of a person's immune system. For Colostrum LD capsules, *"it's suggested to take 1-4 capsules twice daily with 8 oz. water between meals."* The initial dose can be increased to achieve desired results. For children and pets: one capsule one or two times daily. Open capsules and sprinkle into food or drink if swallowing capsules is an issue.

C. Antiviral Supplements

Proteolytic Enzymes

Take Proteolytic Enzymes on an empty stomach, first thing in the morning, and/or at night. They remove the "gunk" from our digestive and circulatory system. They're also therapeutic for herpes, digesting its protective protein layer that surrounds the virus. Eliminating their "armor" leaves the virus unprotected and vulnerable to destruction by the immune system.

Remember, do not take proteolytic enzymes if nursing or pregnant, have a history of ulcers, or take blood thinners. If there is any intestinal discomfort, or discomfort of any kind, back down or stop altogether until the symptoms subside. If in doubt, contact your health care provider to make certain proteolytic enzymes are appropriate for your health.

Lysine

The amino acid L-lysine is recognized as a universal treatment for herpes infections by creating antibodies and disease-fighting cells. While research is inconsistent, many bloggers rate Lysine as effective. However, better results seem to be achieved treating Cold Sores, rather than Genital Herpes. Used regularly, it appears to reduce the frequency and intensity of Cold Sores. It may be worth a try using Lysine for Genital Herpes to see if it helps reduce recurrent outbreaks. If Cold Sores aren't upsetting enough, there's now a growing body of evidence implicating them in the development of Alzheimer's Dementia (AD). http://bit.ly/2E31DsW

Suggested Lysine dose during a Genital Herpes outbreak is:

1. Between 1500 and 2000 mg per day, and
2. 500 mg for daily maintenance.

Try taking Lysine on an empty stomach rather than with food because side effects may include diarrhea, nausea, and abdominal pain. The herpes virus requires the amino acid L-Arginine to replicate properly. Lysine has a similar structure to Arginine but antagonizes its effects, making it difficult for the virus to replicate. Diets rich in Lysine and low in Arginine have been shown to help suppress HSV replication.

Lysine rich foods include yogurt, fish, potatoes, and brewer's yeast. Knowing **L-Arginine** promotes outbreaks, cut back on herpes' *"favorite"* snack foods: chocolate, peas, nuts, and seeds. Lysine cannot be produced by the body and must be consumed in food or supplement form.

BHT (Butylated Hydroxytoluene)

BHT is an FDA approved food preservative and has a long history of benefits against the herpes virus, covered in detail by Mann and Fowke's *'Wipe Out Herpes with BHT.'* Click the link http://bit.ly/2DLXudo to request your free copy. In animal and laboratory tests, BHT proved itself an effective agent against all lipid-coated virus, but there are few human studies. I wonder why?

Many have claimed success using BHT to keep their Cold Sores and genital lesions dormant. Others have had mixed results. Because BHT is a fat-soluble additive, some recommend taking it with coconut oil, while others are just as adamant taking it on an empty stomach. Heavier people need a higher dose. Those with little body fat need less.

A typical dose of BHT ranges from 100 mg - 350 mg once or twice a day with some water on an empty stomach. If it causes stomach upset, try taking it with some coconut oil. A regular multi-vitamin can be taken with BHT, as can L-lysine and 500-1000 mg of vitamin-C. Other than that, it's recommended **BHT be used as a standalone treatment**. High dose vitamin-C is not recommended, and grapefruit juice, colloidal silver, hydrogen peroxide and MSM are also contraindicated.

Side Effects: a common side effect of BHT is dizziness, but *"it may also cause nausea, vomiting, and stomach pain."* Start with 100 mg and increase the dose slowly.

IMPORTANT: do NOT DRINK ALCOHOL while taking BHT. They do NOT mix!

BHT is potent. Careful dosing is required. For those who weigh 125 pounds or less, use no more than 250 mg of BHT per day. For 200 pounds the recommended dosage is 500 mg per day. These are guidelines. A person's age, weight, and fat content also need to be considered. BHT is an over-the-counter supplement, but please consult with your health care provider if you have any health issues or a compromised liver or kidneys. There is a large internet presence of hepatitis patients who use BHT to help improve their disease. Oscar's BHT Hepatitis Treatment www.EarthClinic.com blog can be found here, http://bit.ly/2nr17KQ.

Coconut Oil

Prior to the 1900s, coconut oil was the main dietary fat in the United States. Heart disease was uncommon, and still is in countries where it's widely used.

August 2018, and the American Heart Association (AHA) is still bashing coconut oil via its saturated fat content to reduce cardiovascular disease. The claims made in the AHA report simply don't stand up to the research https://bit.ly/3cfXB33. The AHA continues to reference faulty studies from the 1960s and '70s that saturated fat causes heart disease (it doesn't) and that all saturated fats are the same (they're not). Studies have shown that coconut oil is anti-inflammatory, anti-microbial, and *anti-herpes*. In addition, it may also protect against Alzheimer's disease that HSV-1 is being implicated as a causative agent. So, to sum up the latest coconut bashing propaganda: don't stress about eating coconut oil. The stress is more likely to give you an out-break.

Dr. Bruce Fife is a certified nutritionist, naturopathic physician, and author of more than 20 books, including *The Coconut Oil Miracle* and *Coconut Cures*. He is the director of the www.CoconutResearchCenter.org and represents the southern Colorado chapter of the Weston A. Price Foundation. Even though coconut oil and monolaurin have strong antiviral properties, the question remains, *"Will coconut oil prevent Genital Herpes outbreaks?"* The long and short answer, *"Yes, and maybe."* **TV personality Dr. Oz** did his research. As a result, he dedicated several segments of his show to coconut oil's many benefits. Watch episode number one here http://bit.ly/2Fttl9C.

Treat Genital Herpes and Herpeticum with oral consumption and topical application. Coconut Oil can also be used as cooking oil, butter, and added to that morning cup of *"super"* java. Delicious! The only caution is to build-up internal consumption slowly. Coconut oil has many immune-stimulating and antioxidant properties. It supports thermogenesis (heat) and increases metabolism by nourishing the thyroid and our cells mitochondrial function.

Two factors critical for herpes treatment:

1. Quantity needed to achieve therapeutic levels.
2. How much lauric acid *converts* into monolaurin.

Weston A. Price Foundation suggests eating as much coconut oil as possible to maximize lauric acid levels in the body. Other health advocates recommend starting with two-to-three tablespoons and increasing the dosage www.WestonAPrice.org, until symptoms subside. Results are mixed. Many claim positive results, while just as many have discouraging outcomes. **Dr. Jon Kabara,** credited with discovering the antimicrobial effects of monoglycerides, believes the body converts only a small amount of coconut oil into monolaurin. It may not be enough for a therapeutic response against herpes.

Dr. Kabara asserts the body needs three-to-nine grams of monolaurin a day for an antiviral effect. That's eating 300 to 900 ml of coconut oil a day. I'm not sure if most people want to or even can force down two-to-three cups of coconut oil a day. It might start leaking out their bottom. To get an effective amount of monolaurin, perhaps it's best to take it in supplement form. A single dose of *Lauricidin* is the equivalent of many tablespoons of coconut oil.

What is Lauricidin? The brand name supplement of pure SN-1 monolaurin derived from coconut oil. It was designed to replace large amounts of coconut oil and kill the herpes virus on contact. Lauricidin can also be used as a cream for topical application. Lauricidin is safe and many recommend it. There are thousands of testimonials that claim Lauricidin stopped or greatly reduced their Genital Herpes outbreaks. However, it may need to be taken every day to maintain its effectiveness. There have been no reported negative side effects from long-term use. LAURICIDIN® is more cost-effective when purchased directly from the manufacturer at www.Lauricidin.com.

Lugol's Iodine

Iodine is required by every tissue in our body, but especially our thyroid. It's often called *the endocrine mineral* because of its importance to the thyroid, adrenals, ovaries, breasts, and prostate.

Lugol's Iodine can be used internally or topically on herpes sores. Internal consumption depends on each person's tolerance and deficiency. For Genital Herpes, start with a topical 5-to-10 drop 2.5% Lugol's solution on the inner thighs, sacrum, and/or stomach area. Apply a small dab directly to Herpes lesions once or twice a day. If it stings, dilute with distilled water. Also, unless you're a dolphin or fisherman who only eats seaweed and fish, you're probably deficient. And, if you did decide to eat only fish and seaweed, you'll probably die at a young age from mercury poisoning.

A world iodine deficiency epidemic that probably affects most men, women, and children, but especially vegetarians. Over the past 30 to 40 years, iodine intake in the U.S. has declined by more than 50%, while increasing amounts of competing, toxic halogens of bromine, fluorine, and chlorine have found their way into our food supply. For example, iodine in wheat has been replaced with bromine, the same gas used to fumigate termites in your home.

Most iodine resides in the sea or seashores. So, unless you live in Laguna Beach or Catalina Island, eat fish every day, odds are you're deficient. Other contributing factors:

1. Diets low in fish.
2. Vegan diets.
3. Poor iodine availability in commercial salt.
4. Toxic farming techniques.
5. Avoiding sea-salt for fear of high blood pressure.
6. Ingesting toxic halogens.
7. Radioactive iodine in medical procedures that competes with natural iodine.

Do you have any of these symptoms? Brittle nails, cold hands and feet, depression, difficulty swallowing, dry skin, dry hair or hair loss, fatigue, high cholesterol, hoarseness, infertility, lethargy, menstrual irregularities, early menopause, poor memory or concentration, slower heartbeat, throat pain, weight gain, and yes, frequent herpes outbreaks. If so, iodine deficiency, and/or being hypothyroid might warrant a consideration.

Two forms: iodine and iodide. The thyroid primarily uses iodide. Dr. Lugol's solution is 5% iodine and 10% potassium iodide in water to increase solubility. Two drops of Lugol's 5% solution in water contains about 12.50 mg of iodine/iodide. The Japanese daily iodine intake averages about 13.8 mg, or about 100 times the U.S. RDA. They have lower rates of breast, endometrial and ovarian cancer, and significantly lower rates of fibrocystic breast disease and prostate cancer. The prevalence of herpes in Japan is also far lower compared to that of the United States. Sometimes association is cause.

St John's Wort

St. John's Worth is a strong antiviral substance, so it should be implemented with some degree of caution and on the advice a qualified health care provider that is knowledgeable in natural medicine. There are two options: taking St. John's Wort as a dietary supplement, and/or applying the oil directly to herpes blisters. Both types of St. John's Wort supplements can be found online or at an organic health food store. You can try the recommended dosage for 3 months as part of your Genital Herpes elimination strategy.

Garlic

Numerous studies reported favorable results and therapeutic effects of treating herpes with garlic. Scientists have succeeded in killing the herpes virus in laboratory conditions. The key phrase, "laboratory conditions." http://bit.ly/2DO4gvo **Garlic** contains 33 sulfur compounds, every essential amino acid, all major minerals, several trace minerals, as well as vitamins A, B, and C. But the chemicals allicin and ajoene are what makes garlic effective against HSV-1 or HSV-2. **In 1992, Planta Medica** published a study that used fresh garlic juice on several different viruses, including HSV-1 and HSV-2. Garlic destroyed 90% of any virus within 30 minutes. In their scientific paper, they recommended that people use the following garlic protocol for its antiviral herpetic benefits. http://bit.ly/2nq9U0j

1. **Eat one teaspoon** of fresh minced "raw" garlic every day for prevention.
2. **Eat two teaspoons** at the first sign of an infection.

Allicin is that spicy, scorching, smelly stuff that makes garlic such a powerhouse in a crowded bus or bloodstream. I'm not a big fan of garlic supplements because of their expense, and they don't appear to work as well. A garlic press, some peeled garlic, and a bit of Witherspoon's raw honey and/or organic guacamole may be a better carrier option.

SIDE EFFECTS: according to www.WebMd.com, *"Garlic has been used safely for up to 7 years. When taken by mouth, garlic can cause bad breath, a burning sensation in the mouth or stomach, heartburn, gas, nausea, vomiting, body odor, and diarrhea. Garlic may also increase the risk of bleeding."*

Oregano Oil

For Genital Herpes and Herpeticum

1. Helps prevent outbreaks.
2. Reduces severity of symptoms.
3. Settles down lesions.
4. Protects against fungus and bacteria.
5. Not cheap, but affordable.
6. Suitable for both internal and topical use.

Oregano Oil can relieve the pain and itching of herpes, accelerate the healing process, and prevent spreading the infection. Extracted from the oregano herb, it is an effective free-radical-destroying antioxidant, and a potent antibiotic. Oregano's primary active compound is **carvacrol**. The higher the percentage (85%) of carvacrol, the greater its antiviral properties. It also contains *origanum heracleoticum*, which keeps bacterial strains under control.

Multiple studies, including from the U.S. Department of Agriculture, reported, *"oregano oil has such a strong action against germs that it easily **fights Salmonella and E. coli.**"* One study examined the relationship between oregano oil and harmful organisms and found that taking 600 mg of oregano oil daily prompted a complete disappearance of harmful organisms in the body. http://bit.ly/2FyZiTM

Oregano oil is available in capsule or liquid form. Make sure to purchase a high-quality oil. Some things to consider when evaluating oregano oil. Most oregano oils will contain somewhere between 50 to 85 percent of carvacrol. The more potent, the more expensive.

For topical application it's 'essential' to dilute oregano oil. Some products come pre-diluted (25% oregano oil), but for *sensitive* individuals or children it may need to be diluted further. To dilute 100% oregano, add a "carrier oil." Coconut oil, olive oil, or castor oil are good quality oils. To make a 25% concentration of oregano oil, add 1-part oregano to 3-parts carrier oil. Even diluted, test a small skin area before using it on Genital Herpes sores. It's strong, even at a 25% concentration.

Never use oregano oil or any essential oil in the eyes or ears. If oregano oil inflames the skin, apply more coconut or castor oil, and dilute more. If it accidentally gets into the eyes, add "full-fat-milk" or castor oil to the eye. For internal consumption, dilute oregano oil before swallowing or absorbing it under the tongue. There are several methods to consume oregano oil by the drop:

1. **Hold** oregano drops under the tongue.
2. **Put** drops into an empty vitamin-Capsule.
3. **Mix** oil drops into 2-oz. full-fat milk.

Start with a two-drop dose. It's strong! If you have 25% oregano oil solution, 8 drops of diluted oregano oil will equal two drops of pure oil. The oil can irritate the stomach. Taking it with a bit of coconut oil or fatty food is ideal. There are also commercial gel-cap preparations available on Amazon.

Adding drops of oregano oil to a glass of water is NOT a good idea. The oil will float on top and burn the lips or mouth. It does not dilute or dissolve in water!

There is a surplus of oregano oil. There are also overpriced products sold through personal distributors. While they are of high quality, less expensive but similar oils are available online. Oregano oil offers much when it comes to fighting herpes. Used both internally and externally, it's a safe and effective option to say goodbye and wave bon-voyage to the herpes titanic.

Apple Cider Vinegar (ACV)

If there is a one-word description for the benefits of raw Apple Cider Vinegar (ACV), it would be *"balance."* The gentle way that ACV with "the mother" brings balance to the body is its most important property. But please, use only raw and organic ACV with the "mother." Raw, unfiltered ACV is a fermented food, "like sauerkraut, kefir, kimchi and kombucha. Its cloudy appearance and cobweb strings means the vinegar is living and full of nutrients. The strings are the mother, like kefir grains used to ferment kefir. If there is no mother, there would be no vinegar." www.EarthClinic.com Raw ACV is made from apples and nothing else. They are crushed into fresh apple cider and allowed to ferment.

On the other side of the isle, grocery store vinegars are heated, filtered, and pasteurized. They look sterile and transparent compared to Bragg's Organic unfiltered ACV with the *mother*. Depending on how it's used, grocery store vinegar is OK for some external applications, such as a fungal foot soak. But for internal consumption, please use only organic, raw ACV.

Topical ACV for Genital Herpeticum area; dilute raw ACV with an equal amount of distilled water. Dip a cotton ball into the ACV and dab it on the affected areas three or four times a day. For best results, apply at the first sign or initial tingling sensation. Be aware, it's going to sting, but it'll calm down. The acid in the vinegar quickly goes to work removing excess oil and drying out the sores and lesions. If a 50/50 solution feels comfortable, try a stronger blend the next day until the lesions heal. Repeat until there are signs of improvement.

Internal ACV for prevention. Listed below are several options and protocols:

Breakfast: add two teaspoons of raw unfiltered ACV to a clean glass of water. Consume first thing in the morning before breakfast. This regular health tonic can help strengthen the gut flora and body's immune system, while keeping herpes dormant.

Lunch & Dinner: add two tablespoons of ACV into a 16 oz. empty glass bottle, then mix in ¼ teaspoon of baking soda. Wait until the fizzing stops and fill with clean, pure water. Drink half during lunch, and the other half with dinner. It's best to start low-and-slow with one or two teaspoons and then increase the amount over time. For certain acute conditions, or chronic Genital Herpes outbreaks, more can be taken at any time.

Maybe ACV belongs in your medicine and not kitchen cabinet. But like all treatments, ACV may not be the perfect remedy for everyone. While it works for many, for some it causes side effects. It's OK to start with a lesser amount and increase the dosage slowly until a desired effect is obtained.

Lecithin

Nerves are coated with a fatty insulation called the myelin sheath. This sheath acts like the rubber lining around an electrical wire to prevent interference and keeps the energy flowing. Lecithin may be helpful in preserving the integrity of the myelin sheath and combating the deterioration of the nerve pathways caused by Genital Herpes outbreaks.

Lecithin is a non-toxic fatty compound occurring naturally in animal and plant tissues. Many blogs support the use of Lecithin supplements to stop Genital Herpes outbreaks. In addition, it is said to be useful to control eczema. Hospitals use lecithin-based formula's on newborn babies whose mothers have Genital Herpes.

Anecdotal evidence on many blogs suggest taking between 2000 - 4000 mg a day for thirty (30) days to prevent outbreaks. I recommend a Non-GMO Sunflower Lecithin versus Soy Lecithin. You can purchase Lecithin in powder or gel caps.

D. Topical Antivirals

Essential Oils

Oregano, Clove, Tea Tree, and Myrrh are four popular oils that support the infection healing process. Start with Tea Tree. It has natural antiviral and bacterial properties and can be applied "neat" (undiluted) or mixed with a carrier oil. Or mix and match all four essential oils in various combinations, by either blending them "neat" or with a carrier oil. Experiment and see which combination works best for you. Your three basic options are:

1. **Apply each oil separately** with a Q-tip, or
2. **Blend all four "neat"** (undiluted, without a carrier oil); or
3. **Blend them in a 1 oz. dropper bottle** and add a carrier oil of choice.

For a carrier oil use either coconut, olive, or castor oil. For sensitive skin types, please patch-test oils before using them. Put a drop or two on an inner forearm to make sure there are no negative reactions. Start slow, and if too strong, dilute them further with a carrier oil. Then apply and coat sores three times daily or as needed. Remember, if you use oils 'neat' (undiluted), one-to-three drops is usually sufficient. For the sacrum, you may prefer a 50/50 mix with a carrier oil. For all sensitive skin areas (labia, genital, or lips) consider further dilution. Start slow, then work your way into using them neat.

Manuka Honey

Manuka honey delivers better results than Acyclovir ointment when treating symptoms of labial or Genital Herpes. A good brand is Wedderspoon http://bit.ly/2np8nrh raw honey for treating both Cold Sores and Genital Herpes. Do not use processed sugary, honey found in supermarkets.

In clinical studies, manuka honey effectively eradicated over 250 strains of bacteria, including antibiotic-resistant strains. However, if the infection is serious, like **Herpeticum**, *Medihoney* may be a better choice. *Medihoney* is an advanced wound care dressing that promotes wound healing.

Lemon Balm Antiviral Cream

Lemon Balm Cream is an excellent herbal remedy for the treatment of herpes, blisters, shingles, and Cold Sores. The salve increases the production of skin cells to heal Cold Sores, shingles, and pox rashes. Regular topical use may also lessen outbreak frequency. Amazon has several options to choose from. Review their ratings, stick with those that are "natural" and have a favorable return policy.

Abreva Docosanol Cream

Abreva cream works for Cold Sores by penetrating the skin to the source of the virus. It claims to block the virus and provide a barrier to protect healthy skin cells. It's not intended to be used for Genital Herpes, but some HSV-2 bloggers have claimed success using it. I have no personal experience with Abreva. Click the link below to learn what Abreva users have to say about its effectiveness. http://bit.ly/2GBLYiK

Zinc Oxide, Castor Oil Cream

Zinc helps the body produce lymphocyte cells, which can reduce herpes outbreaks and boost the immune system's ability to fight the virus. Studies show that zinc deactivates herpes and inhibits reproduction. Sores may heal up to 40% faster than leaving them to heal on their own. Zinc can also relieve the pain experienced with outbreaks. A zinc castor oil cream by "Third Day Naturals" is typically applied before bedtime, and overnight the herpes sores can shrink and dry out. If an outbreak is severe, apply the cream intermittently throughout the day, alternating with other options.

The cream is not designed for Cold Sores, but as a barrier cream. However, in test tubes, zinc has been shown to be an effective agent against both HSV-1 and HSV-2. In one small study, people who applied zinc oxide cream to Cold Sores saw them heal faster than those who applied a placebo.

WARNING: Zinc Oxide ointments are recommended for men but not for women in the vaginal area. **Drying agents** should not be used in the vaginal area. Use a Q-Tip or cotton swab to apply Zinc Oxide creams.

Silver Gel Cream

A potent silver gel cream from www.SilverPure.com can be used on herpes lesions, eczema rashes, or Herpeticum infections. The company creates skin creams and salves infused with 35,000 Parts Per Million (PPM) nano-silver particles. There is obviously a difference between 35,000 PPM and the more common drug store 25 PPM, not only in PPMs, but effectiveness. As of this writing, their products do not contain harmful chemicals or skin irritants, only natural oils, mixed with various antioxidants. They are then infused with 10,000 to

35,000 PPM elemental silver nanoparticles, giving the creams powerful anti-microbial properties effective against bacteria, viruses, and fungi.

For thousands of years, silver was the first-line-of-defense against pathogens. Then patentable antibiotics hit center stage. However, unlike with antibiotics, bacteria, viruses, and fungi have not built immunity to elemental silver. Best of all, it's non-toxic.

MMS1 & DMSO Solution

Do a patch test inside your forearm before applying MMS1 or DMSO to your Genital Herpes lesions. Be extra cautious when applying it to the sensitive areas of your privates. Remember, everyone's biology is unique, and we react differently to what we put in and on our bodies. Chlorine Dioxide (MMS1) and DMSO are strong medicine. Treat them with respect.

Topical MMS Solution for Herpes and Herpeticum

1. **Add 4 drops** of un-activated MM, to a glass shooter.

2. **Add 4 drops** of 4% HCL.

3. **Wait 30 to 60 seconds** (it's now activated or MMS1).

4. **Add 4 drops** of 99.99% DMSO to the solution.

5. **Wait a minute and mix with 6 drops** of distilled water.

6. **If the outbreak is severe,** add 3 drops of distilled water.

7. **Use a Q-Tip lightly apply** the MMS1 mixture to blisters.

E. Eczema Protocols

Eliminate

The protocols start by eliminating foods that can aggravate eczema. You may want to consider eliminating:

1. **Citrus Foods**: they contain salicylates and amines which can worsen eczema symptoms for some people.

2. **Tomatoes:** they also contain salicylates, amines, and monosodium glutamate, which can worsen symptoms for many.

3. **Sugar:** reduces immunity and increases inflammation. In addition, it feeds candida and fungal infections.

4. **Dairy Products:** including eggs. Many people are allergic to dairy and can be the cause of "leaky-gut" syndrome. A condition where the gastrointestinal tract becomes porous and "leaks" particles into the bloodstream that shouldn't be there. These may cause an allergic reaction, and eczema.

5. **Junk Foods:** apart from all the toxic chemicals, including MSG (monosodium glutamate) a flavor enhancer which makes food taste better, they do not provide important vitamins, minerals, or nutrition that the body needs to function properly.

6. **Hot Showers:** the number of showers and how hot the water is important for preserving the protective barrier of the skin. Too many showers with very hot water can lead to skin dryness and aggravate eczema symptoms. Keep the water slightly above lukewarm and shower every other day. See if that helps. If symptoms improve you may want to take a European approach, and shower once a week. I know, it stinks, but if it helps resolve eczema who cares. Do a sponge bath.

7. **Alcohol:** for most health conditions, stop. No amount of alcohol is safe for eczema sufferers.

8. **Smoking:** don't!

Start

1. **Sleeping and Resting More:** it is important for health in general, but more so for eczema sufferers because it is critical for regenerating your skin. Sleep deprivation can be a contributing cause of aggravating eczema symptoms and resulting flare-ups. Try to get between 7 and 8 hours of sleep per night—not in the day.

2. **Intermittent Fasting:** this is a favorite of Dr. Mercola to stay or return to health. Not eating for at least 12 hours during a 24-hour period allows the body to regenerate and more efficiently regulate hormones and enzymes. Make sure to consult your doctor if you have any medical conditions such as diabetes before you begin. For example, you may want to eat breakfast at 7 AM (or skip), lunch at 1 PM, and dinner at 6 PM. I eat my largest meal at 6 PM because it allows the body more than 12 hours to assimilate its nutrients.

3. **Probiotics:** the good guys or bacteria of the intestinal tract or "friends of humanity." Without them we suffer. Because of our stressful lives, lack of sleep, and toxic food supply our gut bacteria are under constant siege. To replenish our gut there are a variety of supplements and foods that help to repopulate the intestinal tract. Two of my favorite are Apple Cider Vinegar (ACV with "the mother") and Kefir. Bragg is an excellent ACV brand. The cloudy part is known as "the mother," which includes enzymes, proteins, and probiotics. Simply add a teaspoon, or more, of ACV to 50 ml of Aloe Vera, and enjoy. Kefir is also an excellent source of probiotics. My favorite Kefir is made from goat's milk, which tends not be as dairy problematic.

4. **Water:** be one with water or drink water like a shark. In other words, you're probably not drinking enough. No matter what, more water. It may be your missing link. At least 4 liters or more than a gallon a day. IT'S THE MOST IMPORTANT prescription for eczema.

5. **Exercise:** sweat the eczema out. Some consistent form of exercise 5 days a week that gets your heart rate up so you can work up a sweat. Weightlifting for 20 minutes after jogging, the treadmill, or stair-stepper helps keep your muscles strong. Some testimonials speak of exercise as the holly-grail for eliminating their eczema flare-ups.

6. **Salads:** Salads every day will keep your eczema at bay, but don't forget the chicken breasts or sardines. Along with eating lots of vegetables (cooked), eating a good quality protein every day is important for amino acid content.

Chapter 10: Psychology of Health

Most people become interested in their health only after they've misplaced it. Then they want to quickly find it again. And who can blame them. Herpeticum is out-of-place, an immune system gone astray. Unfortunately, health is not like misplacing your keys or glasses. Quick solutions, instant remedies, or a pill for every ill, often end up exchanging or compounding losses even further. Please don't be like most people. If you've misplaced your health, and are out-of-sorts, be patient, and even if it's lost forever, there are answers that'll help you find your smile again.

So, what is health? Modern medicine tells us when there is no disease, what remains is health. This is deception in the form of a truncated definition. It's like defining light in relationship to darkness, or life to death. If you're not dead, you're alive. Genius. Medicine's dilemma? They are focused on disease not health. The irony, most of the time they don't even know its cause. But they know how to treat symptoms with endless rounds of drugs, chemo, radiation, or surgery. For example, *"Most cancer patients in this country die of chemotherapy. Chemotherapy does not eliminate breast, colon, or lung cancers. This fact has been documented for over a decade, yet doctors still use chemotherapy for these tumors."* Allen Levin, MD, UCSF — *The Healing of Cancer.*

Maybe it's time to change our approach. A good place to start is for doctors to treat the person, and not the disease. We the people need to become more of our own health advocates and Tapping and Meditation is a process toward achieving that goal.

A. EFT Tapping

Emotional Freedom Techniques (EFT), or simply Tapping or EFT Tapping, is a form of psychological acupressure. It's based on the same energy meridians used for over 5,000 years in traditional acupuncture, but without needles. Not only does EFT work, it also has impressive science and research http://bit.ly/2FyTtp0 to back up its claims. Take your physical and emotional well-being into your own hands with EFT. It's simple, effective, and anyone can master it. The best part, it's free.

Tapping provides relief *"from chronic pain, emotional problems, addictions, phobias, Post-Traumatic-Stress-Disorder, and most physical diseases. Like acupuncture and acupressure, the practice consists of Tapping with your fingertips on specific meridian points to release energy blockages."* http://bit.ly/2FAmGAf If Herpes, Eczema, or Herpeticum have you feeling tired, unwell, in frequent pain, depressed, or anxious, consider EFT. Tapping is one of the cornerstones of the Hermes Protocol.

"The cause of all negative emotions is a disruption
in our body's energy system." - Gary Craig

With EFT you "tune in" or focus on the issue while stimulating (Tapping) various meridian points on the body with your fingertips. For most health-related issues, it reduces the conventional therapeutic process from weeks, months, or years down to minutes, hours, or days. Millions have embraced EFT worldwide. Astonishing results have been achieved for pain, diseases, emotional issues, PTSD, and performance enhancement. An original EFT Manual (now obsolete) by founder Gary Craig was translated into 23 languages and downloaded by over 2 million people worldwide. http://bit.ly/2nuOjTW

"EFT is an emotional version of acupuncture,
except we use our fingers and not needles."

Start EFT by learning the locations of the energy points. They're not difficult to memorize. The diagram on the next page illustrates their points in detail. In addition, there are literally hundreds of YouTube presentations where you can simply tap along with whatever issue or subject interests you. Click here http://bit.ly/2E13Wwy for the basic recipe by EFT founder Gary Craig.

EFT works both on an emotional and physical level to improve our well-being. Its intent is to find the root cause of the problem and thereby collapse the "beliefs and negative emotions" that disrupt the body's energy system.

"EFT can assist physical healing by resolving
underlying energetic or emotional contributors."

How a Negative Emotion is Caused

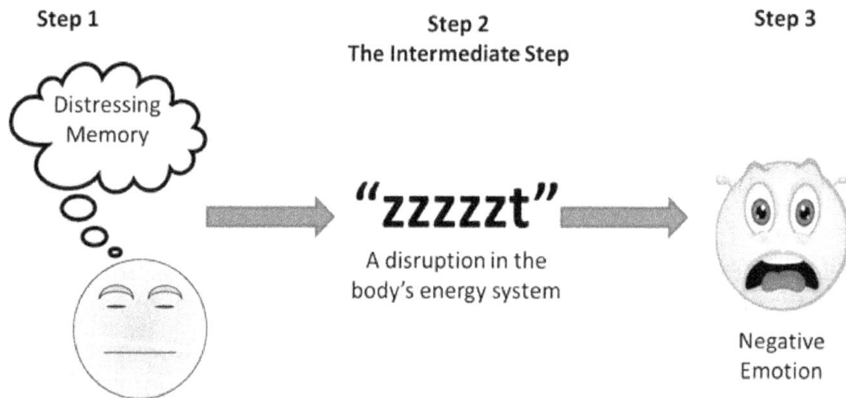

The theory behind EFT is quite simple. *"Deep-rooted emotional wounds are stored in the body/mind as blocked energy patterns. Stimulating specific energy points by gently Tapping on them, while at the same time mentally focusing on them, over time releases their obstruction.*

As the energy is brought back into balance, thoughts about distressing circumstances change, and negative emotions diminish. This process takes place on a bio-electromagnetic level throughout our being."

6-step EFT Tapping Technique

1. **First, Choose a problem.** For example, *"I have an Eczema Herpeticum outbreak on my sacrum."*

2. **Then tune in and rate the intensity** of your negative feeling to that problem, from 0-10 with 10 being the most intense. *"I rate my negative feelings, combined with the pain and discomfort as an 8."*

3. **After rating your intensity,** state the following affirmation three times while Tapping the Karate Chop spot (see the chart of Tapping Points below): *"Even though I have an infection on my sacrum, I deeply and completely, love, honor, and accept myself."*

4. **Tap the remaining energy points** as you speak a reminder word or phrase such as, *"this infection on my sacrum"*, or *"my anger/fear/guilt about my Herpeticum outbreak on my sacrum."*

5. **Take a deep breath.** Take stock. What is your rating now? Notice any new thoughts or memories and repeat Step 4 as often as needed until each one is neutralized.

6. **Return to the original problem** and repeat Steps 4 and 5 until you reach zero or the problem is resolved. Zero means that you no longer feel any negative charge.

Tapping Points

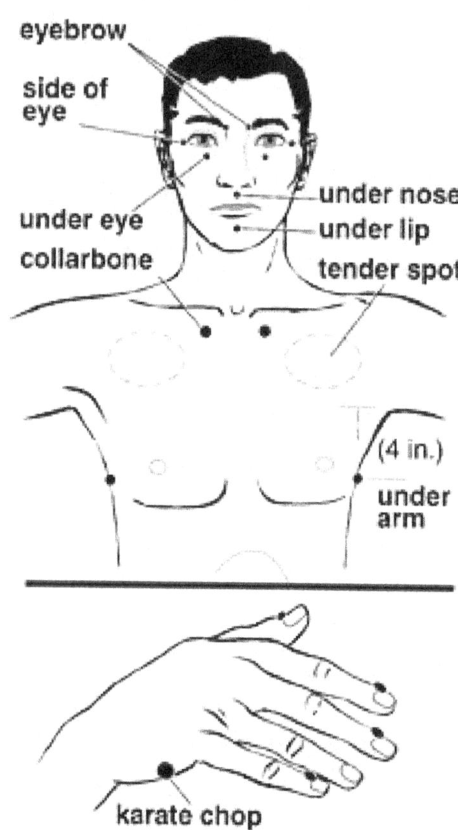

Tapping Points and Their Corresponding Meridians:

1. **Karate Chop – KC:** Small Intestine Meridian – side of the hand, small finger side

2. **BE – Beginning of Eyebrow:** start point of the Bladder Meridian

3. **SE – Side of Eye:** endpoint of the Triple Warmer Meridian, beginning point of the Gall Bladder Meridian

4. **UE – Under the Eye:** Stomach Point Meridian

5. **UN – Under Nose:** endpoint of the Governing Meridian

6. **CH – Chin:** endpoint of the Central or Conception Meridian

7. **CB – Collarbone:** Kidney Meridian & Adrenal Gland Function

8. **UA – Under Arm:** ending point of the Spleen Meridian

9. **TH – Top of Head:** this point (set of points) is located at the top of the head and highly sensitive. Be sure to tap gently on this area, using all your fingers.

EFT can be applied to physical symptoms without exploring an emotional cause. However, for more positive and longer lasting results, it's best to identify and/or target the underlying *emotional issue.*

"Over a million-people suffering through natural or human-caused disasters have been treated with EFT, according to charities that offer aid to these victims." (Capacitar, 2013; TREST, 2010; Veterans Stress Project, 2013). Something to think about when we reflect on those displaced and suffering individuals when Irma and Harvey slammed into Texas and Florida in August and September 2017. Be grateful, seek happiness--not pleasure.

Brad Yates is a favorite tap-along YouTube partner. http://bit.ly/2E5XODk He has a large following and covers hundreds of different Tapping solutions via his website and YouTube Channel.

Listed below are 3 Brad Yates Tap-Alongs:

1. **Optimal Health** - Metabolism and Aging http://bit.ly/2E0TEg1
2. **Healing from the Inside Out** http://bit.ly/2rWA9QS
3. **Happy Tapping** - Clearing Negativity http://bit.ly/2BHw6rf

Gary Craig, the originator of EFT**,** is the consummate teacher and educator. The EFT Dapper-Tapper! The excellence of his training is only surpassed by commitment and contributions to the EFT community. To get up to Tapping speed, visit www.emofree.com. It's Craig's Official EFT Training Center. I started with Gary Craig, and he remains the 'go-to' resource for instruction and technical questions.

1. **EFT Tapping Intro** by Gary Craig http://bit.ly/2DPPIuV
2. **EFT and Emotional Balance,** Gary Craig http://bit.ly/2E2FoTJ
3. **EFT for Serious Diseases,** Gary Craig http://bit.ly/2Fxu2Ep

Nick and Jessica Ortner, a brother and sister team, have written several bestselling books under their main title, *The Tapping Solution*. It's also the name of their website. *The Tapping Solution for Pain Relief* is one of their latest best-sellers.

1. **EFT Tapping for Pain Relief** - Nick Ortner http://bit.ly/2EtTYli
2. **Tapping Meditation** - Love, Peace, & Light: Jessica Ortner http://bit.ly/2nwgOk1
3. **Nick Ortner Taps with a Skeptic** on Shoulder Pain http://bit.ly/2BHUuJ2

B. Medication to Meditation

"The trouble with ignorance,
it picks up confidence as it goes along."

Mindfulness and Meditation

February 2, 2013, the University of Wisconsin-Madison, in the journal of *Brain, Behavior and Immunity,* reported what we've known all along. Meditation reduces the symptoms of many inflammatory diseases. Click here http://bit.ly/2ntTp2E to read the full story.

An ounce of meditation is truly worth a pound of medications. In time, but often later than sooner, most herpes sufferers will do the right thing and try to calm their minds—after they've exhausted most other option. Everyone wants to be rid of "herpes of the flesh," but few are willing to give up their Arginine "pleasures."

Medication-to-Meditation is a part of the Hermes Protocol and a practical guide of mindfulness to achieve wellness. Meditation enhances our ability to:

1. Synchronize the body and mind.
2. Overcome habitual behaviors.
3. Relax within discipline.
4. Face the world with openness, and
5. Without fear.

Disciplined, formal meditation practice might involve each morning and evening, at a specific time and duration. Mindfulness in meditation combines our senses with the mind's attention on any given object. For example, being mindful of the *breath* is a common form of meditation. Following the breath expands consciousness into being fully present in the "Now" moment. But mindfulness can be practiced at any time, not only during meditation. We can use it to be fully present in any moment, no matter where or what we're doing.

Mindfulness, not "thinking-a-mess" may help:

1. Ease the physical symptoms of outbreaks.
2. Calm the mind and emotions.
3. Improve consciousness.
4. Increase compassion toward oneself and others.
5. Develop a sense of love, respect, and acceptance moving forward.

Yes, it can be helpful to take Herpeticum seriously, but not disproportionate to the rest of life. Not to where we're constantly complaining about our *"woe-is-me"* problem. Preferring isolation over companionship and holding resentments against loved ones and acquaintances. And finally resorting to a "bargaining mentality" with God, yourself, and others. *"I'll be good, as long as…."*

"Today I accept personal responsibility
for uplifting my life." - RH

By meditation we mean:

1. Sitting on a chair or cushion.
2. Assuming a good posture.
3. Developing a sense of *"being."*
4. Developing a *"knowing-wisdom."*
5. That you are in the right place and time,
6. Right here, right now.

Meditation allows us to disconnect from our discursive stream of thoughts. However, meditation is not about NOT thinking. If it were, most meditators would be institutionalized or go la-la. It's about observing our thoughts and realizing their transparency by being aware of the deep blue sky that includes them.

Meditation is not an escape but a process of self-awakening. Medication is the language of the flesh and the ego, meditation of the Universe's deep blue sky. It's the prescription into wellness. Instead of coming to meditation with the same "knowing" attitude that has prevailed for most of our lives, we come in an atmosphere of openness. Only to discover who we are at our wisest and most confused, but not making a big deal out of it either. For example, we acknowledge the pain of **Herpeticum**, but we don't make it THE "pain." We learn to respect things without putting the magnifying glass over them. Not belittling, but not fueling either.

Three Elements of Meditation

Choose a spot that's away from the hustle and bustle of daily life, where you'll not be disturbed. Meditate early in the morning. Initially, keep your sessions brief, no more than 5 to 10 minutes.

1. Posture.
2. The object of meditation.
3. How to deal with your thoughts.

Posture: sit upright on a flat surface, either on a cushion or padded folding chair. The feet are planted firmly on the ground with an upright back. Try not tilt to the front, back, or sideways. Feel well balanced. A good posture is important. An upright/straight back is not an artificial posture, but natural. A stiff back is not.

Do not slouch. It makes breathing more difficult. Don't strain by pulling the shoulders up or pushing the chest out. Don't hold the head down, as if bending to something. If sitting on a chair, allow the legs to rest naturally on the floor, hip width apart. Hands resting, palms open, on the thighs. Keep the heart and eyes unlocked by sitting with an open front. Try not to gaze around. Keep the focus slightly downward, about six feet in front of you. Have a sense of belonging and openness. The mouth is accessible, the openness barely visible, just enough to relax the jaw, face, and neck. This also allows the breath to flow naturally. If there is discomfort, make slight adjustments.

Object of Meditation: be mindful of the out-breath. Sit with a good posture. Keep putting the attention on the OUT breath. As you breathe, be fully present. As the out-breath dissolves, the in-breath happens naturally. Then breathe out again, putting more attention on the out-breath. There is a constant going out, flowing in.

Again, and again, keep focusing your attention on the out-breath. As the breath dissolves, the in-breath occurs naturally. No need to follow it. Just keep mindful of your posture, ready for another out-breath. Relaxing, letting go, softening outward, keeping a light awareness of the breath as it goes out. Again, and again.

Working with our thoughts: Oh, no! A thought! It's Ok. Meditation is NOT about NOT thinking. If it were, we'd all get very discouraged. When thoughts arise, we simply and gently say to ourselves, "thinking." Like a feather touching a soap bubble, say to yourself "thinking." Without judgment. Don't say it out-loud. Say it spiritually. Labeling any thoughts with "thinking" gives us leverage to coming back to the breath. It doesn't matter what thoughts we have: whether we have herpes thoughts, negative thoughts, or benevolent thoughts. All are regarded as "thinking." They are neither virtuous nor sinful. Please don't be shocked by your thoughts. Just label them all as simply "thinking," and go back to the breath: "thinking," back to the breath; "thinking," back to the breath.

A Formal Practice of meditation will transition into mindfulness in daily life. As we sit on this earth, eventually a sense of dignity will arise. We start to feel that we deserve this earth and the earth deserves us—with or without Genital Herpes.

Meditation teaches us to be honest and genuine, true to ourselves. The way to liberate the world is to begin liberating ourselves from the "busy" mind and its negative and often exaggerated opinions. From being open and honest with ourselves, we become open and honest with others.

Chapter 11: Overview

The Hermes Protocol is designed to relieve the physical symptoms of Herpeticum, and to exchange our uptight, herpetic-victim-leotards for a peaceful, abiding super-caped-crusader mindfulness mantle. Many of us live our life in a constant sequence of recurring problems. As soon as we're finished with Eczema or Herpes, a problem in a relationship appears. Then another at work, and more unfriends in an unsocial media. And on-and-on-and-on it goes in our "routine existence."

Meditating and Tapping every morning and night reinforces the body's "restorative" powers, opens its meridian channels to a higher, faster recuperative energy. Tapping has never failed to lift my mood, with feelings of awe and respect for the body's healing capacity. Rather than fixating on Herpeticum, and what's wrong, we look for what's right about our health.

The reality is we have a compromised immune system, and herpes will most likely not mystically disappear. But today, through EFT and meditation, we have options to introduce a higher energy Spirit and not turn an outbreak into World War III. Like walking into a dark room, we can turn the light on at any time. Darkness disappears into a light annoyance. Discover the power of turning on the light of life though meditation and Tapping.

Everything is energy. From the food we eat, to the clothes we wear, the cars we drive, and the sun that sustains earth's life. The only difference, they're all vibrating at different frequencies. Slower frequencies appear more solid. This is where our physical problems like herpes show up. Faster frequencies such as light, our emotions, and thoughts are less visible. The fastest frequencies are what Wayne Dyer calls "Spirit." The difference between physical and spirituality is like the inner and outer world. Yes, they are part of "One" world, but *"two unique expressions of being human."*

Everyone is biologically unique. Some are faster, others slower in their recovery. While doing the Hermes Protocol, please be deliberate and steady. This is not a 50-yard dash, but a marathon of getting better one-day-at-a-time. If you feel overwhelmed, stick your head back under the covers. Start afresh. Try different protocol combinations until you find the ones that work best with your immune system and well-being.

Protocols to choose from depend on a person's:

1. State of well-being, disease, special needs, or circumstances.
2. Financial resources necessary for protocols & supplements.
3. Genital Herpes outbreak frequency and severity.
4. Available time to administer and manage protocols.
5. Desire to learn more about each protocol & supplement.
6. Humility to ask for help when necessary.

A. Hair Analysis (HTMA)

Third Reminder: Hair Tissue Mineral Analysis (HTMA) is highly recommended to determine vitamin and/or mineral deficiencies and the body's level of toxins. Please be cautious before starting a supplement regimen prior to your HTMA results. Otherwise, it may compound an already imbalanced profile.

HTMA KITS: can be ordered through <u>www.aurorahealthandnutrition.com</u>, or <u>www.DrLWilson.com</u>. Dr. Wilson has a long list of approved "helpers" to initiate his program.

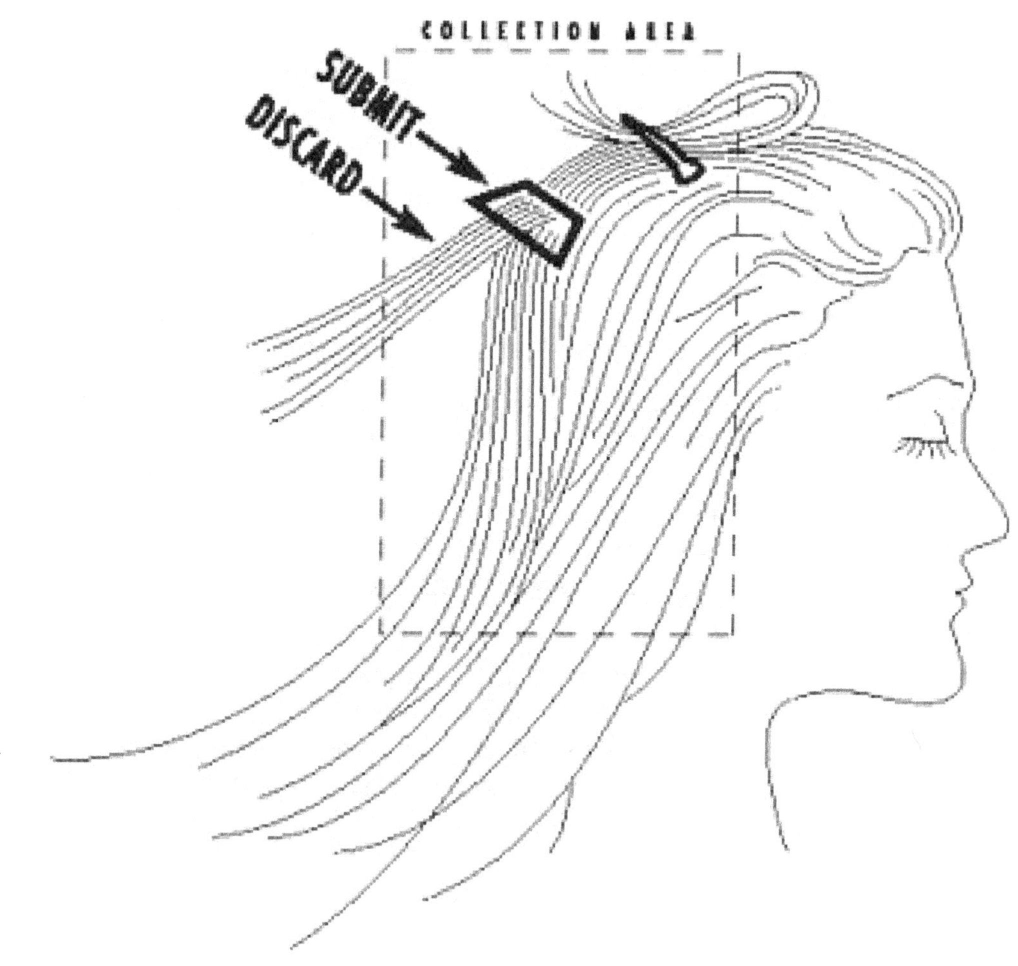

B. Banerji Homeopathy

In hindsight, I would start with the "Banerji" Homeopathic Protocol. But only if you're 100% certain that it's Herpes (HSV-1 or 2) and not some other infection. Instead, it was my last protocol, but with it, chronic Genital Herpes outbreaks stopped in May 2017, and with it Herpeticum dried up and healed.

However, I need to qualify my "outbreak-free" status. Remember, association does not necessarily mean cause. It could be that my Herpes Free condition has more to do with the many protocols prior to undertaking Banerji. These included:

1. **Mineral hair analysis**
2. **Nutritional balancing diet**
3. **High-dose vitamin-C.**
4. **Vitamin and mineral supplements.**
5. **Bob Beck Protocol.**
6. **BHT**
7. **MMS or Chlorine Dioxide.**
8. **Essential oils.**

Was Banerji homeopathy the key after all the other protocols? Your decisions in which protocols and supplements to use, in what order, is largely determined by the results of the HTMA. However, no matter what, start today with a healthy diet. Dr. Wilson's Nutritional Balancing Diet http://bit.ly/2rWOH2Q is one example you may want to consider.

Be cautious when using homeopathy like the Banerji protocol. *"It's real medicine, not to be taken lightly."* www.JoetteCalabrese.com According to Calabrese, *"It is acceptable to give some things a try on a whim, in the hopes it will make a difference. This is not so with Homeopathy. Instead, I urge my students and readers to be absolutely certain of what they are treating." "If what someone believed was Genital Herpes turned out to be jock itch, some other fungal infection or eczema instead, the Banerji protocol… if used repeatedly, could actually cause the symptoms it was intended to remove. It wouldn't cause herpes, but could cause symptoms that might resemble it, that's how Homeopathy works."*

Banerji for HSV-2

1. **Camphor 200,** one dose for one day only. This is used to help clear medications.
2. **Mercurius Solubilis** (or Mercurius vivus) 200c, twice daily.
3. **Arsenicum Album 200c,** twice daily over many months!

According to Calabrese, *"In some cases, improvement is reported within days, while in others, there's simply a lessening of presenting symptoms. Still, others report that the eruptions continue to occur but are less intense, shorter in duration and the episodes are fewer and far between… the speed and depth of this protocol is dependent on such factors as the amount of suppression from drug use in the past, the immunity of the person, and drugs the sufferer may presently be taking.*

Chapter 12: Daily Schedule

*"**Herpeticum is temporary.** It may last a few hours, a week, a month, or even all year. But eventually it will retreat, go back into hiding, and then something else will take its place. But, if I give up and quit, it will last forever. That concession, a final act of hopelessness, stays with me. So, when I feel like quitting. I ask myself, which would I rather live with?"* Author unknown but modified by Reinhard Hermes. I've taken the liberty to change some of the wording to exemplify herpes vs. nerve pain, which can also manifest itself from chronic herpes infections.

The following supplements, vitamins, hormones, medications, and protocols are an interchangeable combination and part of a morning ritual that depended on whether Genital Herpes outbreak(s) were active or not. Remember, the schedule of supplements listed below is a program that the author followed at a specific point in time. There are other combinations that may serve your purpose better. Please consult with a health care professional and wait for the results of your Hair Mineral Tissue Analysis before starting any protocol.

A. Morning

DMSO and MMS

During an active outbreak, after meditating and/or Tapping, but before eating or drinking anything, I take one teaspoon of 99.9% pharmaceutical grade DMSO in 2-ounces of Aloe Vera juice. Then I'd apply a "topical" blend of DMSO and MMS1 to any active lesions.

Mixture Instructions for Sacral Herpes:

1. **Add 5 drops** of un-activated MMS into a 1-or-2-ounce shot-glass.

2. **Activate MMS using 5 drops of 4% HCL** and wait 60 to 90 seconds.

3. **Then add 5 drops** of 100% pure DMSO.

4. **Wait 2 minutes** and add 5 to 10 drops of distilled water.

5. **When ready,** lightly dab it on any lesions.

Caution: Add more drops of distilled water for sensitive skin. Also, make sure to test DMSO for sensitivity or allergy first. Put one or two drops inside the forearm, then three or four. Topical DMSO mixture applications and strengths vary according to past results and experience. Lemon balm or Lysine can also be mixed with DMSO at strengths of 50% to 90% percent, instead of blending it with MMS1.

It's a trial-and-error "sacral" or "facial" (HSV-1 or HSV-2) process to determine the highest concentration that doesn't cause excessive irritation or reddening of the skin. You can add Aloe Vera gel to make the DMSO cream less harsh. The earlier treatment starts, the better results.

Half an hour after taking a teaspoon of DMSO in two ounces of Aloe Vera juice and applying a topical mixture of MMS1-DMSO to any active outbreak, I take enzymes and my Thyroid Meds.

1. ## Proteolytic Enzymes.
2. ## Thyroid Meds with a glass of water.

Proteolytic enzyme deficiencies can contribute to herpes outbreaks by affecting your thyroid health. Proteolytic enzymes, aka systemic enzymes, act as natural immune modulators to help bring the immune system into balance. http://bit.ly/2EsxQYi Taking proteolytic enzymes two hours away from food is like playing the old arcade game Pac-Man. But instead of ghosts, proteolytic enzymes wolf down rubble and debris throughout the body.

Safety and Side Effects: do not take proteolytic enzymes if nursing or pregnant, have a history of ulcers, or taking blood thinners. Also, do NOT take them at least a week before having elective surgery. If in doubt, please contact your health care provider and make certain proteolytic enzymes are appropriate for your health.

Thyroid medications are the second top-selling category of drugs in the U.S. And depending on who you believe, current estimates range between 13-to-27 million Americans have some form of thyroid disease. http://bit.ly/2rYGifo Optimizing thyroid hormones is critical for proper immune function, especially for those who suffer from chronic herpes infections, blood sugar imbalances, sleep disorders, emotional stress, malabsorption issues, or other systemic infections (h-Pylori or dental infections). In short, anything that disrupts the normal state of the body creates hormone imbalances. Until those stressors are dealt with, it is unlikely to experience good health and be "Herpes-Free."

Stress causes the body to release cortisol (adrenal hormone) to douse inflammatory fires. If the body is constantly stressed, it will have chronically high cortisol levels, which can cascade into a blood sugar roller-coaster-ride. As a final insult, stress inhibits the conversion of Thyroid T4 to active T3 hormone. *"Goodnight, and welcome to being constantly tired, immune compromised, and never-ending herpes outbreaks."* Furthermore, decreased T4 to T3 conversion can lower body temperature, dropping immune functions even further, as enzyme efficiency declines.

Hormones are like an orchestra, in that each member plays an "instrumental" role. But, the conductor (thyroid) and his baton (adrenal cortisol), should be synchronized since they arrange and involve most other hormones. *"Not now, trumpets! Slower, violins. Wake-up, kettlebells."*

B. Lunch

Budwig Diet

Lunch is the biggest meal of the day. Besides digestive enzymes, I take most of my vitamins and minerals according to my Hair Tissue Mineral Analysis (see Chapter 11) . Two or three times a week I eat "The Budwig Diet," with two cups of steamed vegetables.

Dr. Johanna Budwig, 1908-2003, a German biochemist, was a seven-time Nobel Prize nominee, and a world-renowned physicist and pharmacist. How German. Dr. Budwig was a persuasive advocate for consuming flax seed oil (The Budwig Protocol) to cure many metabolic diseases. She scientifically connected the relationship between cancer research and fat metabolism. www.budwigcenter.com Based on her extensive scientific research, Dr. Budwig developed a diet that proved successful in treating many metabolic diseases, but specifically cancer. She had an unheard-of success rate, similar to Dr. Max Gerson. Unlike in the good ol' U.S., where most successful alternative cancer clinics have been shut down by the FDA, they continue to flourish in Europe and South America. Many still staunch advocates of Dr. Budwig's cancer diet.

The Budwig Diet emphasizes healthy fats, high antioxidant fresh vegetables, fermented probiotic rich dairy products, sauerkraut, cottage cheese, organic yogurt, flaxseeds, and flaxseed oil. The diet is referred to as the Flaxseed Oil Diet.

Dr. Mercola has continued Dr. Budwig's mission to educate the public on why healthy dietary fat is crucial http://bit.ly/2GBoZnP.

Apple Cider Vinegar (ACV)

ACV helps the immune system, alkalizes the body, kills candida, and keeps Genital Herpes under control. For lunch add two tablespoons of ACV into a 16 oz. empty glass bottle, then mix in ¼ teaspoon of baking soda. Wait until the fizzing stops, and fill with clean, pure water. Drink half during lunch and the other half with dinner. ACV strengthens the gut flora and body's immune system, which will help keep the herpes virus dormant. Start with one or two teaspoons in a glass of water and increase the amount slowly.

For certain acute conditions, or chronic herpes outbreaks, more can be taken at any time. While ACV works well for most, some experience side effects. Start slow and increase the dosage gradually. http://bit.ly/2EsUG1X

The Banerji Protocol

Take before lunch:

1. **Mercurius solubilis** (or Mercurius vivus) 200c, twice daily, and
2. **Arsenicum album** 200c, twice daily over many months.

Take the pellets 30 minutes before or after eating, but best on an empty stomach.

C. Dinner & Evenings

Before retiring for the evening, I take my supplements and medications to boost the immune system in its battle against Genital Herpes and infections:

1. Proteolytic Enzymes
2. DMSO (During an Outbreak)
3. Melatonin
4. LDN (Low Dose Naltrexone)

DMSO and MMS

Repeat the morning procedure during an active outbreak. Take one teaspoon of 99.9% pharmaceutical grade DMSO in 2 ounces of Aloe Vera juice. Apply a *"topical"* blend of DMSO and MMS1 to any active lesions:

Mixture Instructions for Topical Application of DMSO and MMS to Sacral Herpes:

1. **Add 5 drops** of un-activated MMS in a 1 or 2-ounce shot-glass.

2. **Activate MMS** with 5 drops of 4% HCL, wait 60 seconds.

3. **Add 5 to 7 drops** of 100% DMSO.

4. **Wait 2 minutes** and add 5 to 10 drops of distilled water.

5. **When ready,** lightly dab it on any lesions.

Proteolytic Enzymes

Dosage: After the first week, take one capsule in the morning and one at night, preferably 2 or 3 hours after dinner:

1. Keep the dosage at **2 capsules** for the next week.

2. If there is no discomfort, **increase to 3 capsules** a day, in any combination, both in the morning and at night. For example, take 2 capsules AM and 1 PM.

3. **For most, 2-3 capsules a day** is an optimum long-term dose. However, for those suffering from debilitating and chronic inflammation, consider taking one full dose in the morning and another in the evening. (See warnings and side effects under the morning schedule.)

Melatonin

Melatonin regulates the body's internal clock, the sleep cycle. But it carries out a "vast array of other tasks," including regulating certain immune responses (herpes), protecting the body against radiation exposure, and tinnitus. Melatonin supplements cause few side effects but can interact with pharmaceutical drugs. Talk with your pharmacist or health care provider if you're taking any medication to make certain melatonin will not interfere and cause unwanted side effect. I found an interesting small study, *"Regression of herpes viral infection symptoms using melatonin and SB-73 in comparison with Acyclovir."* http://bit.ly/2FxldKX

"The aim of the study was to investigate if 2.5 mg melatonin and 100 mg SB-73 would help patients with herpes, and to compare it to a control group who took 200 mg Acyclovir. SB-73 is a mixture of magnesium, phosphate, fatty acids extracted from Aspergillus, which has anti-herpes virus properties. Almost 96% of the melatonin patients reported a complete regression of symptoms after 7 days of treatment. By comparison, 85.3% of the Acyclovir group reported regression of symptoms in the same period. There was a statistically significant difference between the groups."

A book by Jeff T. Bowles, *Extreme Dose!* Melatonin the Miracle Anti-Aging Hormone is a good alternative resource to learn more about Melatonin's benefits. Bowles has been known to take LARGE amounts (up to 500 mg) without side effects, other than sleeping 14 hours a day.

Dosage: I've personally taken 3 mg to as much as 50 mg a night, but never more than not waking up refreshed. If groggy and sleepy in the morning after taking melatonin, it may be too large a dose. Build up slowly. My last supplements before going to bed are **melatonin and 3 mg of LDN.** The do not seem to interfere with one another. Like MMS, and vitamin C, there are also a lot of melatonin warnings about consuming more than 3 mg. Read Jeff Bowles book on melatonin. He has the research and personal clinical experience to offer more than biased propaganda. In Europe, melatonin is used as an adjunct for birth control at a dose of 75 mg a night. http://wapo.st/2nskCnf

LDN (Low Dose Naltrexone)

LDN is an "off-label" medication approved by the FDA and used frequently by "alternative" doctors to treat autoimmune diseases. Taken at bedtime, LDN works by briefly blocking opiate receptors and "tricking" the body into increasing endorphin production. Endorphins are a vital part of a healthy immune system that LDN facilitates to correct immune defects. One of the first patent applications was for the use of LDN in HIV herpes infections. Elaine A. Moore, *"The Promise of Low Dose Naltrexone Therapy,"* (p. 104), Kindle Edition. Up-to-date information about Low Dose Naltrexone (LDN) for patients, physicians, and researchers can be found at www.LDNScience.org.

Dose and Frequency: It is generally recommended to begin with 3.0 mg per day and adjust the dosage if necessary. Prescribing 1.5 mg capsules allows easy adjustment. For example, the patient can take either 2 capsules for 3 mg, or 3 capsules for a 4.5 mg dose. I've taken a 3 mg dose at bedtime for almost 7 years.

Side Effects: **LDN has virtually no side effects.** During the first week, some patients report vivid dreams, and others occasionally complain of difficulty sleeping. If this persists after the first week, dosage can be reduced from 4.5 mg to 3 mg. LDN is virtually non-toxic, simple to administer, relatively inexpensive considering it's not insurance approved—about $50 per month. Good night and sleep melatonin, LDN well.

D. Detoxification

Instead of being in constant conflict with herpes or eczema, let outbreaks and rashes motivate us to untangle and transform our perceptions of life's many disappointments. That way we'll be better prepared to face those of the future.

Herpeticum is like a sword, frequently wounding and scarring relationships, and cutting through our illusions. As we look at our life, as it represents itself in our hearts, can we accept the truth? That to live with or without herpes or eczema, is to experience pain, joy, sorrow, happiness, loss, and grief. It's all part of the human condition that we all have in common. A much bigger problem than herpes or eczema is for those who can't see or feel that. Unintentionally making them in constant conflict with life itself.

Just as sadness can be the wellspring of creativity, happiness the fountain of authenticity, so can Herpeticum be the motivator for peace of mind.

The conscious mind controls the brain only 5% of the time. I thought, "No way!" My mind is like a jumping flea. Giving it 5% was kind. I'm kidding, but it's very believable that the subconscious controls our thoughts 95% of the time. http://bit.ly/2DRm5K0

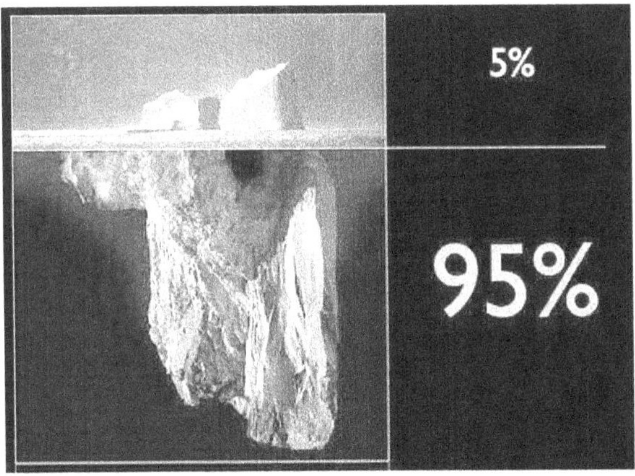

Detoxify or Acidify

It's important to wash your car before detailing it. Emptying the trash before replacing it with a new liner. Taking off soiled sheets before putting on clean ones. Showering after a workout before stepping into clean underwear. And *not over-supplementing in advance of detoxifying;* otherwise, all desired outcomes can be contaminated.

The ER physician first stops the bleeding, just as the Hermes Protocol aims to first improve chronic herpes infections and eczema rashes. Our goal is to leave the ER on our own accord. To have the immune system keep us Herpeticum free without constant intervention. So, take the trash out, and reestablish immunity.

Today, everyone, including newborn babies are toxic and mineral deficient. It's disturbing to find more than 200 chemicals in African American, Hispanic, and Asian newborns. *"The study focused on minority children to show that chemical exposure is ubiquitous. Building on 2005*

research on cord blood taken from 10 anonymous babies.” http://bit.ly/2rYX8e6
IMPORTANT: Wireless technology is a physical health hazard. Its addictive use is a precursor to mental infertility and emotional immaturity.

Like cancer rates, electromagnetic pollution is getting worse, not better. To the point that today everyone is toxic. It only comes down to how heavy a load. Newsflash: toxins cause untold suffering and sickness, the cruelest of which is malignancy. People who feel tired all the time may just be carrying a heavy toxic load. Like driving an overloaded dump truck with a burned-out dashboard and the emergency brake on.

Most lab values are like automobile dashboards. They don't tell you anything unless something is already broken. Otherwise, why do we see so many stranded, overheated cars, hooked up to a tow-truck? They started okay that morning. Their *“smart-dashboard”* said, *“All is well.”* Even though it wasn't. When your doctor looks at your labs, they see a “normal” reference range, taken from a bunch of overweight, toxic, unhealthy people, who were advised to do bloodwork.

“Normal ranges” are calculated so that 95% of *“healthy”* people have values that fall within the normal range. The catch-22 is the word *“healthy.”* We all know how healthy most people are. If you want to be like them, then let the “all-is-well” lab values be your guide.

Supplements and Procedures to help detoxify:

1. **Detoxify the Liver.** It's the first and most important organ of detoxification, followed by the kidneys and our skin. There are several first-rate liver protocols but start by improving your diet. Then take some extra supplements to help detoxify.

2. **Eat Cruciferous Vegetables.** Even though they're goitrogenic and a problem for some hypothyroid patient, they support healthy liver function and its phase 2 detoxification. If you're hypothyroid but iodine sufficient, then eating normal amounts of cruciferous vegetables shouldn't be a problem.

3. **Eat Garlic.** Allicin in garlic helps detoxify the liver. As side benefit it keeps Genital Herpes in check. See Chapter 11, Antiviral Supplements, for more information on the benefits of garlic.

4. **Cilantro** may help remove heavy metals and is commonly included in certain detoxification products.

5. **Chlorella** is often called a super-food and may help remove heavy metals such as cadmium and mercury. It can prevent the accumulation of dioxins within the body and be beneficial for liver cancer patients.

6. **Milk Thistle** is one of the most popular herbs to protect and improve liver health. It may even prevent the formation of gallstones. Silymarin is the active ingredient that protects the liver and kidney cells from the toxic effects of drugs.

7. **Globe Artichoke** is an herb that is useful for liver toxicity or damage. It can also help improve bile production.

8. **Dandelion** is another herb to help to improve liver function.

9. **Schisandra** is one of the highest antioxidant berries to improve the detoxifying capacity of the liver, both for acute and chronic liver diseases.

10. **Infrared sauna therapy** is beneficial in eliminating toxins, improving circulation, and reducing blood pressure. Many well-known healthcare professionals recommend using sauna therapy, including Dr. Mark Hyman, Dr. Joseph Mercola, and Dr. Lawrence Wilson. Although many realize the benefits of infrared sauna therapy, there is a difference in opinion when it comes to near vs. far sauna therapy. Some endorse infrared sauna; others favor far infrared sauna. Both are beneficial. Most units sold are far infrared saunas.

11. **CAUTION:** many herpes sufferers have a love-hate relationship with the sun, sweating, and sweltering heat. If Genital Herpes breaks out with every fever, a day at the beach, or from sweating every time you work out, skip the sauna until the predator is back in its box.

12. **Activated Charcoal** is made from bone char, coconut shells, peat, or sawdust. Its medical use dates to Hippocrates (400 B.C.) when physicians treated epilepsy and anthrax with it. After the development of the charcoal activation process (1870 to 1920), reports appeared in medical journals about its use as an antidote for poisons and intestinal disorders. Porous and negatively charged, it helps bind a variety of toxins, preventing them from being absorbed into the body.

   Activated charcoal is ordinarily considered safe, but for some it can cause unpleasant gastro-intestinal side effects. If you have any medical conditions such as intestinal bleeding or blockages, recent abdominal surgery, then activated charcoal may not be for you. Please check with your doctor. Activated charcoal can interfere with the absorption of nutrients, supplements, and prescription medications. Take activated charcoal 90 minutes to two hours prior to meals, supplements, and medications. Always check with your healthcare provider if any of these conditions apply before taking activated charcoal.

Cleanse the Colon

There are numerous ways to cleanse the colon. If you go online, or walk into any local health food store, there is no shortage of kits or supplements to cleanse the colon.

Coffee Enemas: Dr. Max Gerson's promoted coffee enemas to detoxify the liver, increase glutathione production, and eliminate pathogens. As a side benefit, they cleanse the colon. The other advantages of coffee enemas? They are done in the privacy of your own home and are extremely cost effective. My initial reaction at a Max Gerson seminar <u>www.Gerson.org</u> was, "What?" Sorry, but I take my espresso through the esophageal tube, not my sphincter. Despite my initial suspicion, by the time I finished the seminar and looked at the science, I decided to try them.

It took a while to overcome the mental resistance. But the first time I heard that all familiar gall-bladder "squirt," and my temperature went back to normal, I quickly saw their benefit. Dr. Wilson's website has complete details on how to go about taking a coffee enema. http://bit.ly/2BKgsv9

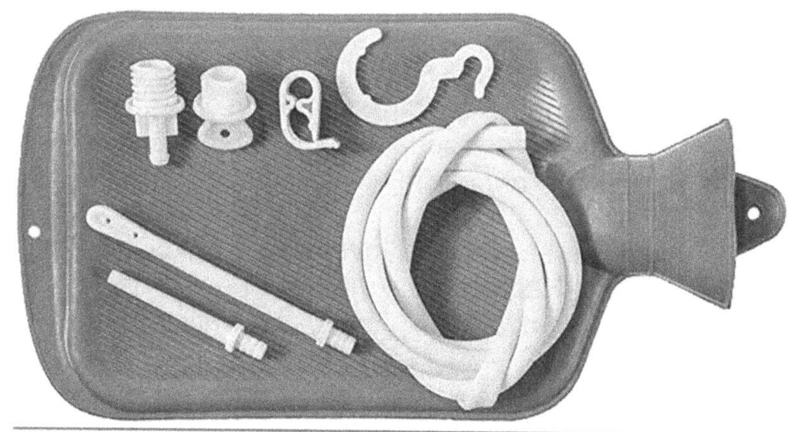

Enema Colon Kit

Colon hydrotherapy and colonic irrigation are other methods to clean out the colon. For colon hydrotherapy/colonic irrigation it's best to see a certified hydro-therapist. The advantage of colon hydrotherapy is that it does a better job of cleansing when compared to coffee enemas. However, for some people, it is too aggressive. For example, if someone has increased intestinal permeability (a leaky gut), then it's probably best to refrain from colon hydrotherapy.

Whatever method(s) you decide to use, consider a liver-kidney-colon detox program to support the immune system in its efforts to keep Genital Herpes dormant. Finally, detoxification is not a 100-yard dash, but a New York marathon. Start all doses and protocols low and slow. Work your way up. Try not to do too much all at once. Detoxing will take anywhere from 30 days to several months. Sometimes longer. Also, pulse your treatments on and off. Otherwise, they'll lose their effectiveness.

Water Warning: don't underestimate the importance of drinking and using purified water in your home. The worst offender is fluoride. Unlike chlorine, fluoride is not eliminated by boiling water. The best solution is to install a kitchen sink and shower filter that removes fluoride. Or purchase bottled water in gallon jugs and make sure it contains no toxic chemicals.

Knowledge is power, *but excessive knowledge weakness.* If you decide to use the Hermes Protocol (HP), do your research. Well-informed advocates make better choices. But, once you decide, stay the course until you're Herpeticum Free.

The Hermes Protocol can be intensive, expensive, and at times overwhelming because of its life-style changes, supplements, treatments, and mind-therapies. But as Thomas Jefferson wrote, *"The price of freedom is eternal vigilance."* Well, so is the price of Herpeticum **Freedom.** If you falter, pick yourself up. Brush off the temptation to quit before the miracle happens. Get back on the diet, adjust your supplements, get back into meditation, and trust your inner voice. If you're still uncertain, ask for help.

Chapter 13: In Closing

It is my sincere hope that you have found solace and relief with the Hermes Protocol. Remember, it's key to cleanse the body and purge the mind of gloom. Then unlock the body-mind connection, as we let go of our negative emotions.

Thank you for your efforts in looking for a permanent solution, rather than a quick fix.

I believe the Hermes Protocol's mental approach to physical health challenges will benefit any situations. If you have questions or concerns, please feel free to contact me at rhermes1@gmail.com, and I will respond as quickly as I can. Now for a few final observations.

Healing the sorrow of Herpeticum does not occur through blame or judgement, or by being in denial. It's the willingness to discern without judgement. To see life as it is, so we can live openly in truth, no matter what. Eventually, we come to realize that "My Friend, the Enemy," is not only Herpeticum, but us.

That's often hard to own, but don't be afraid. People who have gone through personal tragedies, the loss of a loved one, divorce, cancer, combat, and PTSD, say that what got them through was thinking back to a time when someone loved them unconditionally.

Whether it was a wife, lover, Mom or Dad, or an old uncle, who saw them and knew who they were, and loved them without conditions. Even if it was just for a moment.

Yes, inside that space of time they knew love and felt lovable. It doesn't take much, just one person in one moment. Maybe it's time to extend that mercy to ourselves. While at the same time getting over the fixed idea, "My life should be a certain way, but especially without Herpeticum." We don't control life's ingredients, only what we do with them.

So, no matter what physical or mental problems we experience, instead of getting anxious and fearful, sit back, relax, and be as still as possible. See their reality and try to understand what can be done. Yes, the real solution to Herpeticum is to face it first. Then try and understand the infection through our wisdom, not fear. If we do that, most of our difficulties will fade with time, or just disappear.

Shift our small eczema and herpes story, into a more open agenda. Realize that even though they are not our friends, they are also not the enemy. It's just life.

A. Peace for Happiness

Acceptance is the key to healing and transformation. Acknowledging to yourself that chronic herpes outbreaks and eczema flare-ups can be a common occurrence for a compromised immune system. And that there is nothing inherently "wrong" with us is the first step in the healing process. What it does, it takes away the guilt and shame that surrounds it. Denial is a common defense mechanism we use, pretending herpes or eczema is not a big deal. Until it turns into one, Eczema Herpeticum.

Accepting the state of our body, including Herpeticum, is to be proactive instead of inactive and wishful. Embracing our sickness, changes our entire emotional construct into a more calming and soothing state of mind. Make peace with your herpes or eczema history. Our biggest spiritual growth takes place on the back of difficult burdens. Take hold of Herpeticum, even if you need help, and turn it into just another hurdle and ingredient along your journey.

What we're really doing is *embracing the truth and reality of our life* instead of pushing it away. In that embrace we find a sense of ease, an understanding that we may never have a perfect, healthy body, and that the one we have is good enough. With that approach we engage our body instead of rejecting it. With engagement comes a feeling of peace. And with peace we begin to realize that we don't have to change who we are. Only when you accept and honor your history will you retire the "enemy" gracefully. Accept all chapters of your life story. Allow the lessons of Herpeticum to make you stronger.

With feeling "right" about ourselves comes freedom. Freedom to be who we are and to make the most out of the life we have. Instead of listening to our faultfinding mind, with its constant selection of negative thoughts spotlighting our defects and those of others, we can instead have the appreciative mind. The kind of mind that embraces our faults and the character defects of others. Embrace our wisdom that accepts the life we experience. With acceptance something else happens. Often our health improves. Outbreaks and rashes are diminished as we acknowledge the pain, instead of trying to reject it.

It's the negativity that we give to our experiences that's the real problem. The lack of tolerance creates more tension, stress, guilt, and pain. And the endless desire to escape our experiences, wishing things were different causes more suffering. If we accept our condition, part of the disease and stress is removed. And even though antivirals often alleviate herpes outbreaks entirely, it's the mind and our thinking that respond to acceptance and love. Not Valtrex. Stop making eczema the enemy. Embrace and make peace with it, and in the process, free yourself.

For those who already meditate, you know the more you try to control the mind and your thoughts, the more problematic the practice becomes. We never get still in meditation by trying to be still. The way to stillness in meditation is to care for the mind with the same compassion and love we tend to our children. In meditation we stop arguing with ourselves, our mind, or our heart. We make peace with every moment. *The real source of happiness is inner peace.*

B. Fear to Confidence

*"I've learned over the years that when one's mind
is made up, this diminishes fear; knowing what
must be done, does away with fear." - Rosa Parks*

For us to experience peace and happiness, it's essential to transcend fear into confidence. Fear takes many forms with Eczema, Herpes, and Herpeticum. From the shock and panic that comes over us when we first break out or test positive, to the emotional challenges that confront our relationships.

There are countless strategies we use to take our mind away from or off our diseases. Some drink. Others do drugs. A few meditate and practice yoga. Many seek refuge in TV or bury themselves in romantic novellas. The adventure types go to a local pub and have a few beers. Anything but be alone with our anxious mind. But eventually some of us get fed up with our repetitive routines and boredom sets in. With boredom we are closer to fear.

If we hide out from the world, we may feel more secure and think that we've quieted our fear, but all we've done is make ourselves numb. Surrounded with our habitual thoughts, a "cocoon" environment, we hope nothing else will harm us. Afraid of our own fear, we have walled off our hearts.

As we experience our sadness, gradually we come to realize that maybe Herpeticum isn't the enemy. Maybe it's our mind. Perhaps if we start to make friends with ourselves by being more human, gentle, and open, we can change. Not the feeble, milk-and-honey gentleness, but a basic goodness kind, from which we gain strength and confidence. Confidence that doesn't come about through self-improvement but in aligning the body and mind to thrive together. In their harmony we alleviate our fears.

For example, the body can be compared to the camera in your iPhone. The mind is its film or memory chip. The question is how to use them together to get a clear, accurate picture of our world. Only if the aperture, shutter speed, and memory chip are aligned, can we take good photos. Similarly, when the mind and body are properly synchronized, we get a more accurate, unblemished picture of our world. Without blurry shortsightedness, we begin to trust ourselves and have less fear.

Instead of being ashamed of ourselves, in who we are, our jobs, finances, relationships, education, and our mental shortcomings, we begin to synchronize the mind and body to connect to the world with confidence. This process affects how we see ourselves. Most of all, we don't apologize for being born. As we experience the goodness of being alive, we begin to respect who and what we are through the lessons of Herpeticum.

In working with the Hermes Protocol, cleaning up our life starts with telling the truth. Then we begin to open our heart that fear closed. There is no longer any room for cowards. We shed any hesitation about being honest with ourselves because it feels unpleasant. Cleaning up our past restores our basic goodness and brings us ever closer to confidence, peace, and happiness.

There is no perfection in life. Everything is transient, so expect distress and setbacks from time to time. Learn from your mistakes so you can prevent them in the future. And remember, no one owes you. Also, do not wait for tomorrow or other people to rescue you. Instead live in peace and confidence today.

I want to thank you again for buying and then reading *My Friend, The Enemy* all the way to the end. If you have time, I would appreciate it if you could leave a review. It would help in many ways. Thank you,

Reinhard Hermes, MS

C. Hyperlinks for Eczema Herpeticum

Page 1   https://bit.ly/3HRCM9I   Masks-for-All COVID-19 Not Based on Science

Page 6   http://bit.ly/2DVWCIWiki   130 Herpes Viruses in mammals, birds, etc.

Page 11   http://bit.ly/2BzYnjn   Valtrex Approved 1995, Acyclovir 1982

Page 11   http://bit.ly/2rHWIZk Acy   Acyclovir Studies

Page 11   http://bit.ly/2BAnVNI   Valtrex Studies

Page 11   http://bit.ly/2niNQEY   Acyclovir Studies

Page 12   http://bit.ly/2DVvZgEFamvir Allergic Reaction

Page 19   http://bit.ly/2DGThDD   Viral and DNA Blood Tests

Page 23   http://bit.ly/2E9bZFp   Eczema in early life

Page 25   https://bit.ly/3nAhEvt   Eczema Treatment Phototherapy

Page 25   https://bit.ly/3P6xeuF   Eczema Psychological Counseling

Page 27   https://bit.ly/3yDNuOm   Hand, foot, and mouth disease (HFMD or HFM)

Page 28   http://bit.ly/2DJI35r   Herpeticum Infection Can Quickly Spread

Page 28   http://bit.ly/2DJXdnl   Timely Treatment is Critical

Page 33   http://bit.ly/2Gqd9wl   Herpes Infections 50% are over 50 years old

Page 33   http://bit.ly/2rHykqE   HSV-1 and Mental Impairment

Page 34   http://bit.ly/2EhRupV   Association: Microwave Radiation and Cognition

Page 34   http://bit.ly/2DH8jJD   Herpes Online Support Groups

Page 36   http://bit.ly/2GsMMX4   Social Medial and Feelings of Isolation

Page 36   http://amzn.to/2BBVJcJ   *"There's a Spiritual Solution to Every Problem"*

Page 38   http://bit.ly/2GrkEne   Immune System Malfunctioning

Page 38   http://bit.ly/2GsVaFN   Significant Delay in Healing

Page 39   http://bit.ly/2DYSMZn   The Effects of Thyroid Hormone on HSV-1

Page 41   http://bit.ly/2BBeEEG   IOM Water Recommendation

Page 45   http://bit.ly/2DYimxy   Dr. Lustig Interview About Food Companies

Page 47   https://bit.ly/3bRHRD4   Barbara Frederickson Positive Emotions Researcher

Page 47   https://bit.ly/3NXIoAW   Exercise Effects Immunity (Also on Page 54)

Page 49   https://bit.ly/3Rogil9   Hair Tissue Mineral Analysis (HTMA)

Page 50   http://bit.ly/2np6HOT   Dr. Bob Beck Talks Micro Pulsing and Healing

Page 53   https://bit.ly/3c7Pl5j   CDC Antibiotic Resistant Infections

Page 53   http://bit.ly/2noM1pb   Silver Nanoparticles Inhibited the AIDS Virus

Page 54   http://bit.ly/2nqtSr8   Drug Companies Plot to Regulate Nano-Silver

Page 58   http://bit.ly/2Eembel   Dr. Robert Hill and DMSO Eyesight Study

Page 58   http://bit.ly/2DLHS5G   DMSO and Shingles

Page 59   http://bit.ly/2FvUyhv   Vitamin C for Herpes Infections

Page 59   http://bit.ly/2DWR6iS   Herpes, Shingles, and Vitamin-C

Page 60   http://bit.ly/2EryXaV   Dr. Klenner and Vitamin-C Safety

Page 62   http://bit.ly/2GxjOVV   Latest Cancer Research and Vitamin-C

Page 62   http://bit.ly/2DMpOs0   Low Dose Naltrexone (LDN) HIV and Genital Herpes

Page 62   http://bit.ly/2EoosVO   LDN Impact on Immune System YouTube Video

Page 64   http://bit.ly/2Gsx91E   History of the Genesis II Church

Page 63   www.quantumleap.is   MMS Documentary

Page 63   http://www.wpsuppliers.com   Approved "Water Purification" Vendors

Page 63   www.mmsnews.is   Jim Humble's book: MMS Health Recovery Guidebook

Page 64   http://bit.ly/2rRLQrW   Protocol 1000 (YouTube Video No Longer Available.)

Page 66   http://bit.ly/2no3te8   YouTube terminated MMS Account. I wonder why?

Page 64   https://jimhumble.co/bookstore   Jim Humble's Bookstore

Page 67   http://bit.ly/2GuC42k   No Deaths from Supplements

Page 68   http://bit.ly/2npiCv2   Thymic Protein A to Offset Nutrient Deficiency

Page 69   http://bit.ly/2nqXQvb   Dr. Julian Whitaker, Nutrition Review

Page 69   http://bit.ly/2DQTatC   Colostrum-LD

Page 70   http://bit.ly/2DYBUSi   Colostrum Research